NURSING
MEMORIES
FROM PROBATIONERS
TO PROFESSORS

EDITED BY PAT STARKEY

Gwyneth McLane
Lunchy date
Feb'y 17th 1998 at the
Albert Dock.

NATIONAL MUSEUMS & GALLERIES
· ON MERSEYSIDE ·

British Library Cataloguing-in-Publication
Data Available

© The Board of Trustees of the National Museums and
Galleries on Merseyside, 1994

Published by the National Museums and Galleries on
Merseyside

ISBN 0 906367 67 0

Printed by Birkenhead Press Limited, 1 & 3 Grove Road,
Rock Ferry, Birkenhead, Merseyside L42 3XS.

CONTENTS

ACKNOWLEDGEMENTS

Preparing this book has been a team effort. As each chapter was produced, the working party discussed, criticised and suggested alterations to it. Finally, though, some tidying-up had to be done and I must thank my colleagues for their generosity in allowing me to make changes to some parts of their text, and for their firmness in telling me when they thought that I had gone far enough. We all owe many thanks to Adrian Allan, who, as well as contributing to the volume, has acted as convenor to the group. Meticulous care to detail has characterised all that he done for us and my task as Editor has been made much easier as a result of his efficiency, and willingness to check material and hunt down sources. I thank him particularly for his help in checking the copy and preparing the Index.

We record our thanks to the executors of Mrs Gwen Hardy's estate for the grant given to help with the costs of publication. Gwen Hardy's death was a cause of great sadness to the working party. She had made a major contribution both to the exhibition at the Merseyside Museum of Labour History, and to the working party preparing this volume, and had hoped to include in it the results of the research on which she was engaged when she died. That work, on a register of probationer nurses for 1862-88, is still unfinished.

We also acknowledge the generous grants from the Eleanor Rathbone Charitable Trust and Ocean Group plc (P. H. Holt Trust) which have enabled us to publish this work.

Pat Starkey
University of Liverpool
September 1993

ILLUSTRATIONS

Cover: A selection of nurses' badges from Liverpool hospitals

Page

Permission to reproduce photographs has been given by the
following: 1, 2, 5, 6 and 7, National Museums and Galleries on
Merseyside; 4, Liverpool Record Office; 8, Miss Gwynneth
Rowe; 11 and 13, the University of Liverpool Archives; 12, 14
and 15, Miss Helen Brett; 17, Mrs Betty Hoare; 18, Liverpool
Daily Post and Echo; 19, Photographic Service, Faculties of Arts
and Social and Environmental Studies, University of Liverpool;
20 and 21, Department of Nursing, University of Liverpool; 22,
Simpsons Photographic Service, Liverpool.

NOTES ON CONTRIBUTORS

Mr Adrian Allan read Modern History at the University of Durham and gained the Diploma in the Study of Records and Administration of Archives at the University of Liverpool. He worked as Assistant Archivist, Bury St Edmunds and has been Assistant Archivist at the University of Liverpool since 1970. He has a particular interest in sources for health care history, serving on the Archives Committee of Liverpool Health Authority and, in 1981-82, directing a survey of hospital records and artefacts in the Mersey region. He is co-director, with Dr Starkey, of the oral history project of which Professor Morle is Director.

Miss Helen S.Brett trained at the Liverpool Royal Infirmary and became a committed theatre nurse. In this capacity she served on a number of committees and advisory bodies both locally and nationally, for which services she was awarded the MBE in 1976. She retired in 1986 as Acting Director of Nursing Services at the Royal Liverpool Hospital.

Mrs Winifred Froom's training at Mill Road Infirmary, Liverpool -which commenced in 1938 - was interrupted by the bombing of the hospital during the war, when staff were dispersed. Her general training was completed at Walton Hospital, and followed by midwifery at Smithdown Road Hospital (now Sefton General), ophthalmics at St Paul's Eye Hospital and training at the Queen's Institute of District Nursing. This was followed by marriage, motherhood and the relative obscurity of domestic life.

Miss Mavis Gray trained at the Liverpool Royal Infirmary and gained the Sister Tutor Diploma at Queen Elizabeth College, the University of London. From 1962 she held various posts as Principal Nursing Officer (Education), prior to her appointment as Director of Nurse Education, Wirral School of Nursing, a post from which she retired in 1987.

Mrs Betty Hoare trained at the Liverpool Royal Infirmary and gained the Sister Tutor Diploma from the University of London and a B.A. from the Open University. She has worked in London,

Liverpool, Birmingham and Switzerland and, at the time of her marriage, was Principal Nursing Officer (Education) at The United Liverpool Hospitals' School of Nursing.

Professor Kate Morle trained at the Liverpool Royal Infirmary and gained an M.Sc. in Nursing from the University of Manchester. She became the first Professor of Nursing in the University of Liverpool in 1988. She is Director of a project funded by the Wellcome Trust entitled 'The history of nursing in an English urban region from 1919, based on establishing an oral history archive'.

Miss Gwynneth Rowe trained at the Royal Liverpool Children's Hospital and St Thomas's Hospital, London, and obtained a Diploma in Nursing from the University of London. She returned to Liverpool in 1972 as Principal Nursing Officer, Paediatric Division, becoming Divisional Nursing Officer with the Liverpool Area Health Authority in 1974. She is now retired.

Dr Pat Starkey trained as a nurse at the Nuffield Orthopaedic Centre, Oxford and the Radcliffe Infirmary, Oxford. She read History at the University of Liverpool and now teaches part-time there and at Chester College. She is co-director, with Mr Allan, of the oral history project funded by the Wellcome Trust, of which Professor Morle is Director.

Ms Marij van Helmond worked as a social worker both in the Netherlands and in Britain. After several years in community development and adult education she made a mid-life career change and has been working as a social history curator with the National Museums and Galleries on Merseyside since 1987.

Chapter 1
Nursing Memories
Pat Starkey

We already know a great deal about the main developments in the history of nursing. Brian Abel-Smith, for example, has described the ways in which the profession has developed since 1800: the work of the untrained nurse of the nineteenth century; the struggle for the registration of nurses in the early years of the twentieth; the recruitment of young women to undertake training, and the different, often conflicting, ideas which contributed to the evolution of an agreed educational programme. [1] Rosemary White has discussed the implications for nursing of the establishment of the National Health Service in 1948.[2] Christopher Maggs has highlighted the way in which the trained general nurse came to occupy the pinnacle of the nursing profession.[3] Robert Dingwall, Anne Marie Rafferty and Charles Webster have enlarged our knowledge of the social history of the profession.[4] And Celia Davies and those who contributed to *Rewriting Nursing History* have given us insights into a variety of aspects of the profession, from the role of women healers in past centuries to the ways in which knowledge of nursing and nurses may be gathered from a variety of archival sources.[5] Monica Baly, too, has taken the long view and described the place of nursing in social change from the sixteenth century.[6]

But important though such studies are, most have examined structures and institutions. To date, little has been written about the experience of being a nurse. This collection of essays, therefore, sets out to do two things; to describe aspects of the profession from the point of view of those who have been members of it, and to suggest ways in which our knowledge of nursing could be enlarged by the study of local records as yet unexamined. The impulse for the book came from an exhibition on nursing and nurses entitled 'Ministering Angels? The History of Nursing in Liverpool' mounted by the Merseyside Museum of Labour History in 1989, and described in the essay by Ms Marij

1

van Helmond. [7] Having collected and displayed artefacts from the hospital wards of the past, borrowed old photographs and hospital badges, and jogged the memories of those who had been employed as nurses, the organisers of the exhibition became aware of the lack of any careful account of the experiences of nurses and of the wealth of historical material that had yet to be recorded. This prompted the setting-up of a working party to collect information about nursing and nurses in and around Liverpool. Its first project, a short-term study interviewing and recording the experiences of women who nursed in the city earlier this century, has uncovered valuable information, and its success has helped to attract funding from the Wellcome Trust for more substantial research. But the members of the working party, several of them retired, senior nurses, were also made aware of the value of their own memories in building a picture of nursing in Liverpool and were persuaded to write about them. This publication, largely produced by those nurses, is, therefore, consciously a local study, although the national context is not forgotten.

Few who write about the history of nursing can resist the temptation to draw on those figures who have informed the stereotypes. It is a truism to note that the public perception of nurses has been bedevilled by images fostered by fiction; the alcohol-swilling Mrs Gamp created by Charles Dickens or the harassed heroine of *One Pair of Feet*, described by Monica Dickens, descendant of the nineteenth-century novelist, for example, both describe women who might have been representative of some nurses at some time in history; but they were also created to make political points and to entertain. The more up-to-date, but equally fictitious, stars of the BBC television series *Casualty* bear more likeness to the hospital staff familiar to the second half of the twentieth century; there, nurses are seen taking responsibility for the care of patients, performing procedures like the insertion of sutures and acting as equal colleagues to the doctors. But the programme's slant, which appears to aim at exposing the plight of the National Health Service in the 1990s, and its frequent reference to financial stringency and changes in management structures, sometimes skews the series and detracts

2

from the reality of day-to-day life in a modern hospital. In its way it is just as distorting as any other fictional representation. Television's insatiable demand for drama tends to give a false impression of hospital life: it gives an inadequate account, for example, of the occasional tedium - even in a casualty department - and the reality of relationships between junior and senior members of staff. In what sense is Charlie Fairhead typical of the 1990s male charge-nurse? And are hospital porters and senior medical staff really on such friendly, first-name terms? And what are we to make of the fact that, although most nurses are women, in a popular television series the most senior nurse is a man? Does this represent the real position in nursing hierarchy in modern hospitals, or is another socio-political point being made?

If fiction can misrepresent so can journalism. The 'ministering angels' myth, still perpetuated by some tabloid newspapers, fuels an image of young women - usually beautiful young women - in caps and aprons, with scarcely a technical thought in their celestial heads or little more than soothing skill in the hands used to stroke fevered brows: an image which bears litle relation to the reality of modern nursing. By allowing nurses to tell their own story, this volume treads a path between the academic interests of historians and sociologists and the romantic pictures of novelists, dramatists and journalists.

Adequate training separates Mrs Gamp from today's nurses. Although nurse education received some attention from medical men and hospital administrators, in the nineteenth century hospitals designed and taught their own courses and awarded their own certificates; there was no nationally recognised standard of competence. The struggle to introduce a national Register of trained nurses in the early years of the twentieth century focused on the status of those who were to be allowed to use the title 'nurse' and was, of course, closely related to training (a discussion which, as Mrs Hoare points out, was by no means over in the 1930s).[8] Already a complex issue, and made more so by the arguments of competing factions, progress towards the compilation of a Register was compounded by the events of the First World War. Then the need for staff in both military and civilian

3

hospitals resulted in large numbers of volunteers - mainly from the upper social classes, and organised into Voluntary Aid Detachments - giving their services in hospitals and convalescent homes both at home and abroad. These volunteers received short courses of training, but were perceived as 'unprofessional women'[9] by nurses who had learned their craft in hospitals in peace time; and in the move towards the Nurses' Registration Act of 1919 great efforts were made to ensure that VADs were kept off the Register.[10] But it was not only the status of untrained amateurs which occupied the thoughts of those campaigning for proper recognition for nurses. Christopher Maggs argues that even within the ranks of trained nurses a hierarchy of training developed, and he has demonstrated the way in which general hospital training became the doorway through which all nurses had to pass, with subordinate status being accorded to other disciplines such as fever nursing, children's nursing and tuberculosis nursing.[11] Nurses might qualify in these disciplines either before or after their general training, but on their own they were not sufficient to allow the nurse to progress far in her profession. In the years after the Second World War, nurse education continued to receive attention from the General Nursing Council and the Ministry of Health, and by 1958 the rigid barriers which had grown up between the different parts of the Register began to be relaxed, so that it became possible to undertake a course of training which qualified a nurse for inclusion in more than one part of the Register. By this means a nurse might, for example, undertake a combined general and mental nursing training, or one which included a children's nursing qualification as well as general registration.

Professor Kate Morle's study of educational developments in nursing in Liverpool shows how rapidly changes in nurse training have occurred and suggests advances which are only just around the corner, with graduate nurses now able to register for higher degrees and to initiate research. [12] To some extent Kate Morle embodies the progress made in the second half of the twentieth century. Having trained as a student nurse in the conventional way - by completing a three-year theoretical and practical training in the Liverpool Royal Infirmary - she then studied for an M.Sc. at the University of Manchester, taught in the Department of Nursing at the University of Liverpool, and became its first Professor of Nursing in 1988.

Such dramatic changes as have occurred in nurse training must have their effects in the working environment, and the new breed of highly educated nurses may sometimes cause confusion in the network of relationships in hospitals, traditionally characterised by clearly defined hierarchies. Although the experienced ward sister, who diplomatically advised and guided junior - and not so junior - doctors in the care of patients, was frequently a feature of hospital life, it is only in recent years that nurses with university degrees, and the consequent confidence in their own intellectual abilities, have worked in the wards. The inevitable challenge to traditional relationships may be illustrated by one graduate nurse who, when treated by a junior doctor as though she was both stupid and insignificant, announced that she felt she wanted to pin a badge to her apron saying 'I have a good honours degree - probably as good as yours'.

It is this tension, inherent in a profession which has traditionally expected its members to play 'the doctors and nurses game', which is identified by Helen Cohen. The nursing culture, she argues, internalises two powerful contradictions, subservience and professionalism: the former assumes a readiness just to obey while the latter demands judgement and the ability to put judgement into action.[13] The tension cannot be divorced from the fact that nursing has been, and still is, largely a female profession and attitudes towards nurses have been at one with attitudes towards women. Furthermore, its members have traditionally worn a uniform which owes more to servant clothing in the nineteenth century than to the garb of a highly technical occupation in the twentieth. It remains to be seen whether the slow abandonment of caps and aprons, while mourned by some who treasure their association with particular training schools, will help to alter the image of nurses, not just in the public mind but in the status accorded to them by other members of hospital staff.

There is little that is new in these observations. As Dirk Keyzer has argued, nursing has tended to carry all the hallmarks of a female occupation: limited access to education, high turnover of staff in the clinical area, subservience to the predominantly male occupation of medicine and a career structure limited to management.[14] The origins of the relative lack of status enjoyed by modern nurses in Britain is located by Rosemary White in the shortage of nurses in the period from the beginning of the Second World War when, in an attempt to recruit large numbers of nurses as a matter of urgency, entrance requirements for training were significantly reduced; and to the Ministry of Health's low regard for nurses, illustrated in the Notes for the Guidance of Hospital Management Committees in 1948, where they were assumed to be only slightly higher in status than domestic staff.[15]

But perhaps we should look further back than the 1940s for the identification of nurses with domestic staff. That pioneer in women's education and contemporary of Florence Nightingale, Emily Davies - founder of Girton College, Cambridge, the first college to give women a university education - took no interest in the education of nurses and believed that it was work unsuitable for middle-class women. Writing in the 1860s, she stated: 'The business of a nurse is in every way too nearly allied to that of an upper servant to be in the least appropriate for the daughters and sisters of the mercantile and professional classes.'[16] And Emily Davies was not alone. Elizabeth Garrett - who trained as a nurse at the Middlesex Hospital in the 1850s, before going on to take a degree in medicine at the University of Paris - while allowing that middle-class women might choose to become nurses, also identified the way in which class determined the sort of nursing they might do. In a paper read at the National Association for the Promotion of Social Science in 1866, she argued that head nurses were 'skilful, experienced and kindly people...usually from the lower section of the middle class' while under-nurses were 'vastly inferior...commonly below the class of second- or even third-rate domestic servants; if they were not nurses, one would expect them to be maids-of-all-work, scrubs or charwomen.'[17] Is it possible that we see the legacy of this class bias in the ways in which women were directed to particular schools of nursing according to their educational, and therefore, class background during the first half of the twentieth century?

As Marij van Helmond demonstrates in her essay,[18] those educated in grammar schools tended to apply to the more prestigious voluntary hospitals, while their less fortunate colleagues were more likely to be accepted in the municipal (ex-workhouse) establishments.

The crisis of identity experienced by some nurses in the late twentieth century is itself a mark of the increased confidence of the profession in its own competence. No such crisis would have afflicted a hospital nurse in earlier generations: it was assumed that the doctor was all-powerful and his word could not be challenged. A nurse rash enough to question his decisions would quickly learn that such insubordination would not be tolerated. But although conscious of their low status in relation to the medical staff, the authors of the essays in this volume also depict a profession in which women exercised considerable power and carried great responsibility. For all the deference accorded to the predominantly male medical staff, there is the clear impression that the hospital was perceived by the nurses as a female environment: the significant figures were women. Matron, the departmental and ward sisters, home sister and the sister tutors were more important in the lives of probationer nurses than medical consultants, even though the latters' periodic ward rounds necessitated much tidying of counterpanes and straightening of bed-wheels. The same preparations were made for Matron's daily round, and it was her disapproval that the nurses feared. It is interesting to wonder whether the consultant on his rounds ever noticed whether the openings of pillow cases were facing away from the doors, the bed-wheels were straight, or the sheet on the bed was positioned with the 'right' side next to the patient. Matron would notice. But the rigid nursing hierarchy and strict discipline had positive features. As one retired nurse observed, at a time when there were few women doctors and even fewer male nurses, the senior nurses she encountered during her training invited her respect because of their experience, but also provided her with role models of successful women in responsible posts.

If nurses' experience on most wards was of working with other women, this was less the case in the operating theatres.

7

There they would have closer contacts with doctors than in any other department. But even in the theatres, women were to be found in positions of authority and responsibility. Sister's word was law - at least to the nursing and ancillary staff - and few junior doctors would have dared risk her displeasure. Theatre nursing is, as Miss Helen Brett opines, a child of the mid-twentieth century, and the theatre nurse, as assistant to the surgeon and administrator of the theatre suite, plays a very different role from that of her predecessor, the man who cleaned the room and furniture, oiled the instruments and held down the hapless patient. [19] The past half-century has seen, in this specialised area of nursing as in most others, rapid advances resulting from improved medical knowledge and surgical techniques as well as greater sophistication in the sterilisation of instruments and dressings. Nowadays, the hazards posed by dangerous materials are better understood and Health and Safety legislation exists to protect those who work with them. No nurse in the 1990s would be required to sit for an hour threading radium needles with her bare hands, as Miss Brett did in the 1950s.[20]

One specialism which, when combined with general nursing, could win students admission to the General Register after a four-year training, was that of caring for sick children. Historically, hospitals had been reluctant to admit children: as Brian Abel-Smith has pointed out, some, like the Radcliffe Infirmary in Oxford in 1770, deliberately ruled against having them in the wards.[21] The first hospital in Britain specifically for the care of sick children was founded in Liverpool in 1851; the Great Ormond Street Hospital in London was opened the following year. Miss Gwynneth Rowe paints a picture of the rigid routine which was followed in the children's hospital in the late 1930s and early 1940s, and which severely limited possibilities for visiting; in the years before psychologists such as John Bowlby, writing in the early 1950s, suggested that maternal deprivation might cause damage to the emotional development of children. It is almost as though the instinctive knowledge of the mid-eighteenth century had been lost until the mid-twentieth. Although their tendency to succumb to infection was one reason for hospital authorities wanting to keep children out of their wards,

8

another was articulated by Dr George Armstrong, founder of the first children's dispensary in 1769: 'It very seldom happens that a mother can conveniently go into an hospital to attend her sick infant ... if you take away a sick child from its parents or its nurse you break its heart immediately.'[22]

In the days before the establishment of the National Health Service, hospitals were funded and managed in a variety of ways. But wherever they trained, whether in a municipal hospital or a voluntary one, nurses developed great affection for their training schools and wore their hospital badges or distinctive uniforms with pride. A function of this pride in the hospital was the evolution of the Nurses' Leagues or Guilds, organisations run by and intended for graduates of the schools. From the records of the Liverpool Royal Infirmary Training School Nurses' League, Mrs Betty Hoare has reconstructed the history of one such League. Its purpose was manifold: at one level, it enabled nurses who had trained and worked together to keep in touch with one another and to meet at the Annual Reunion on the third Saturday in October every year. But it also functioned as a means of forging links with similar Leagues, both in this country and internationally, through the International Council of Nurses, set up in 1899 - thanks to the energetic action of the nursing pioneer Mrs Bedford Fenwick - and the National Council of Nurses of the United Kingdom, founded in 1904.[23]

If fictional stereotypes are an almost invariable element in any discussion of nursing history, descriptions of the conditions under which nurses used to work rarely escape mention either. Frequently reference is made to the strict discipline which governed nurses' lives and to the length of their working day. A speaker at the first meeting of the Liverpool Royal Infirmary Training School Nurses' League in 1933 spoke of her experience of training earlier in the century and recalled that she was given her first day off duty after ten months of working on the wards.[24] Things had obviously improved by the time that she was regaling her younger colleagues with tales of the horrors of the past, but nurses in 1933 still worked for 112 hours a fortnight on day-duty and 126 hours a fortnight on night-duty. It was not until 1943 that

9

the Rushcliffe Committee urged the implementation of a ninety-six hour fortnight on as many hospitals as could put it into practice as possible. Hours might have been reduced, but the assumption was still made that the nurse's time was the hospital's to control. A nurse might not know until the 'change list' was read out at breakfast-time that she was to go on to night-duty that evening, and, in spite of the twelve-hour stint of duty that 'nights' entailed, she was still expected to work on the ward until 2.00 p.m. that day. The fact that she might thereby miss her day off for that week was not taken into account when the duty-lists were made up.[25] Rules about time off did not apply at Christmas and in many, if not most, hospital wards staff were expected to work throughout Christmas Day without any off-duty. Miss Mavis Gray describes the festivities at the Liverpool Royal Infirmary, where the celebrations were a long time in preparation and small traditions, built up over the years, were rigorously adhered to. And rigid though they must often have seemed, hospital regulations were sometimes relaxed a little at Christmas to allow needy Liverpudlians to enjoy the warmth of a ward bed and a traditional turkey dinner.[26]

With so little free time, it is not surprising that the hospital environment provided both professional satisfaction and a substitute family for nurses. Mavis Gray attributes to the Liverpool Royal Infirmary characteristics of a normal family, expecting that it would care for its members as a family might. [27] And Mrs Froom's description of the nurses' home where she lived while doing her district nurse training also provides evidence of a female community which provided for both the social and professional needs of its members. [28] But in this area, as in others described in this book, substantial changes have taken place. Now nurses frequently live in their own flats and houses, instead of Nurses' Homes. Hours of work have been steadily reduced. A forty-four hour week was introduced for hospital domestic and ancillary workers in 1957 and the following year the Whitley Council, the body responsible for nurses' pay and conditions under the National Health Service, recommended to the Minister of Health the introduction of an eighty-eight hour fortnight for nurses.[29] In the 1990s, nurses work a thirty-seven and-a-half-hour week. Such changes mean that nurses are no longer almost totally dependent on the hospital community for company and friendship.

The experience of the Liverpool Working Party over the last two years has demonstrated that there is much nursing history to be discovered. From his considerable knowledge of relevant archives Mr Adrian Allan has compiled a list of primary and secondary sources relating to Liverpool and its region in both local and national collections.[30] A detailed study of these will clearly increase our knowledge of nursing in the region. But, as Marij van Helmond points out, documentary sources are not the only ones available to us in our quest for the past, and we neglect at our peril the experiences of nurses themselves.[31] The award of a grant from the Wellcome Trust, and the appointment from 1993 of a Research Associate, will make possible the compilation of an oral history archive of nursing history in Liverpool and its region; the reminiscences of those who trained and worked in Liverpool hospitals will help to put flesh on the bones of our understanding of health provision and life in hospitals.

Notes

[1] Brian Abel-Smith, *A History of the Nursing Profession* (London, 1960)
[2] Rosemary White, T*he Effects of the NHS on the Nursing Profession, 1948-1961* (London, 1985)
[3] Christopher Maggs, *The Origins of General Nursing* (London, 1983)
[4] Robert Dingwall, Anne Marie Rafferty and Charles Webster, *An Introduction to the Social History of Nursing* (London, 1988)
[5] Celia Davies (ed.), *Rewriting Nursing History* (London, 1980)
[6] Monica E.Baly, *Nursing and Social Change* (2nd edition, London, 1980)
[7] See below, pp.13-28

[8] See below, p.89

[9] Abel-Smith, *A History,* p.86

[10] Ibid., p.99

[11] Maggs, *Origins,* passim.

[12] See below, pp.102-7

[13] Helen Cohen, *The Nurse's Quest for a Professional Identity* (California, 1981)

[14] Dirk M. Keyzer, 'Challenging the role boundaries: conceptual frameworks for understanding the conflict arising from the implementation of the nursing process in practice', in Rosemary White (ed.), *Political Issues in Nursing* (London, 1988), vol.3, p.96

[15] White, *The Effects of the NHS*, ch.13

[16] Janet Howarth (ed.), *The Higher Education of Women. A Classic Victorian Argument for the Equal Education of Women* (London, 1988), p.189, n.6

[17] Candida Ann Lacey (ed.), *Barbara Leigh Smith Bodichon and the Langham Place Group* (London, 1987), pp.443-444

[18] See below, p.25

[19] See below, pp.74-5

[20] See below, p.82

[21] Brian Abel-Smith, *The Hospitals, 1800-1948* (London, 1964), pp.13-14

[22] Ibid., p.19

[23] Abel-Smith, *A History*, p.76; Baly, *Nursing*, p.155

[24] See below, p.88

[25] See below, p.49

[26] See below, p.60

[27] See below, p.55

[28] See below, p.34

[29] Abel-Smith, *A History*, pp. 250ff.

[30] See below, p.114

[31] See below, p.16

Chapter 2
Nursing on Show
Marij van Helmond

In February 1989 the Merseyside Museum of Labour History in
Liverpool presented a temporary exhibition entitled 'Ministering Angels? - The history of Nursing in Liverpool'. This
contribution describes the why and how of this exhibition and
explores the problems involved in representing an essentially
modest profession in a museum.

The Merseyside Museum of Labour History in Liverpool was
established in 1986 by the now defunct Merseyside County
Council with the explicit aim of representing the history of the
'ordinary' people of Liverpool. Staff were given just six months
to put the permanent galleries together. Clearly in such a short
period only the main chapters of local people's history could be
researched in terms of material evidence, that is objects and
images for display. Topics such as religion, health and welfare,
and popular culture had to be left to one side. The histories of
specific groups and communities within the Liverpool population were just touched upon and only marginally more could be
shown about women's lives. Subsequently, staff set out to 'fill
the gaps' by means of a programme of temporary exhibitions
with the intention of making the new material thus collected part
of permanent displays at a later date. There were temporary
exhibitions on women's work and on the Anglo-Chinese, Jewish
and Black communities. There was also a temporary exhibition
on health care in Liverpool before the National Health Service.
[1] This latter exhibition prompted two retired nurses to suggest
that there should be a permanent display on the role played by
nurses in the development of health care in Britain. Although a
project of such sweep was outside the remit of the Museum [2], a
temporary exhibition on nursing in Liverpool seemed most
appropriate, not least because of the pioneering role of Liverpool
in the development of the nursing profession. A working party

was formed consisting of the retired nurses, who were joined by a third; an amateur local historian with a keen interest in nursing history; the assistant archivist of the University of Liverpool, and the museum's social history curator. This group met a number of times over the period of a year to discuss the aims and format of the project and to advise the curator on the interpretation of material collected and to comment on draft texts.

The aim of the exhibition was to be two-fold: to present to visitors the important role played by Liverpool in the development of nursing (a 'Liverpool pride' exercise) and, importantly, to represent the women who had made this role possible - the nurses themselves. This was not a simple task as nursing as a profession has developed in a complex way over a long period of time. Its history has been written from a number of perspectives, as Pat Starkey points out in her introduction, but mainly with a national remit. Few, if any, local histories of nursing have been produced so far. Histories of local hospitals or of medical specialisms, yes, but not of the development and experience of nursing in a local context. [3] Yet the development of nursing in different cities in Britain may well have followed different routes, and research into and documentation of such routes must add to our understanding of national developments. For example, was it merely a coincidence that home-nursing for the poor, later to become known as district nursing, was 'invented' in Liverpool?

The next thing to decide was how much of this complex history could effectively be covered by a modest-sized exhibition and what, within the chosen parameters, were to be the key areas. For example, where to start? The 'Florence Nightingale and all that' starting point used in conventional historiography did not seem appropriate, despite the fact that the good lady had a direct input into Liverpool developments. It was decided instead to preface the story with a brief reference to nursing before the establishment of formal training and to take a significant local initiative as the real starting point: the development of a home-nursing service to the poor, established in 1862. [4] The advent of the National Health Service in 1948 would provide the cut-off point as the exhibition could not do justice to its impact on the nursing profession. Therefore the period to be covered by the exhibition

14

would be 1862 to 1948 - more or less. In terms of geographical area, the exhibition would restrict itself to Liverpool's current postal district boundaries, even though local health care provision has not always operated within these boundaries. Liverpool's mental hospitals, for example, were situated well outside the city. As key areas, the group initially identified training; nursing as a career for women; the organisation of the profession; specialisms; nursing during wartime, and social life.

Having decided on the subject for the exhibition, the group discussed available evidence and how to turn it into an accessible and informative display.

The work of Gwen Hardy on the early days of nurse training and district nursing (in Liverpool inextricably linked) turned out to be an invaluable source. [5] However, little research seemed to have been undertaken and published on subsequent hospital nursing practice; the position of nurses in the different (voluntary and municipal) hospital hierarchies; career choice opportunities; pay and conditions; life in the nurses' homes, and least of all, on nurses' own experience of their chosen profession. Adrian Allan, a contributor to this volume, offers future researchers a comprehensive list of available sources,[6] but when the working party started its work no such valuable guidance was available. The listings of archival and other material connected with hospitals held in Liverpool Record Office do not readily reveal material of relevance for nursing history. A good deal of district nursing material can be found under that heading in the sheaf catalogue but for information on school nursing or midwifery more imaginative detective work is required. As with researching other aspects of women's history - which is what nursing essentially is - archive lists and indexes tend not to be very informative. A good working knowledge of hospital organisation and administration goes a long way when trying to figure out under what headings, other than 'nursing', its history may be found.

Research into the experience of nurses themselves, particularly in the early days, is further hampered by the nature of the sources.

15

For example, the early development of district nursing in Liverpool can be traced through a wealth of documents: printed annual reports; reports from Lady Superintendents and minute books of the Select Vestry and the workhouse hospital committee. This history is in Liverpool firmly connected with the person of William Rathbone the sixth, a local merchant and philanthropist who provided the initial funding for the service. But what this material does not provide is information about the woman who gave Rathbone the idea for such a service in the first place. She nursed his sick wife at home so effectively that it made Rathbone reflect on the benefit of such a service to the poor in Liverpool, who had no access to decent hospital care. It was she who undertook a trial project in home nursing, but other than her name - Mary Robinson - we know nothing about her. Equally, we know very little about the actual experience of the first generation of district nurses. Recently a rich source of personal data has become available through the identification of the first registers of the Liverpool Royal Infirmary Training School and Home for Nurses, and their analysis and interpretation promise important insights into that experience, albeit from a perspective other than their own. [7] What can be said about nineteenth-century sources also goes for more modern ones, as hospital records do not record the experiences, views and attitudes of nursing staff. The only sources immediately at hand for this are retired and working nurses themselves. In our case, the retired nurses on the working party willingly dipped into their own memories to give a personal gloss to the more impersonal facts. The value of this particular source, however, was somewhat limited by the fact that all three nurses had spent most of their working lives in the same hospital. First-hand information on the experience of nursing in Liverpool's other hospitals was not available from within the working party. This demonstrated forcefully the need for concerted oral history work if the experience of another generation of nurses was not to go the same way as that of their predecessors - lost in the mist of time.

If literary sources presented a problem, the situation was worse with regards to the material culture, objects and artefacts related to nursing. The Museum possesses only a few items - a small and disparate number of objects and some photographs. Perhaps the porcelain bedpan manufactured in Liverpool or a plaque from a local hospital ward could be given more meaning when placed in a specific context, but they had obviously not been collected with local nursing history in mind. Collections at the University of Liverpool also lacked nursing artefacts and the Liverpool Medical Institution, a long- established professional institution with a considerable collection of books and some medical instruments, could not offer much either. Surprisingly, Liverpool Record Office possesses a cache of Liverpool nursing badges, whilst the Royal Liverpool Hospital has some delightful objects related to the early days of the Liverpool Training School for Nursing. They included a set of brass lanterns used on ward rounds, a framed letter from Florence Nightingale to the nurses of the Liverpool Training School, and some photographs.

The difficulties encountered in the process of collecting suitable material caused the working party to consider more carefully what kind of objects could be seen as specifically connected with or representative of the nursing profession. Were they instruments and items of equipment, and if so, which ones? Was it possible to point at instruments identified with nursing in the same way as stethoscopes or scalpels were with the medical profession? How can notions such as 'care' and 'commitment' and 'discipline', so inextricably linked with nursing, be represented by objects?[8]

It soon became clear that even objects apparently straightforward in nature could be interpreted in more than one way. For example, it was agreed that items of uniform should figure prominently, for several reasons. Over the period in which nursing developed from merely an activity which supposedly 'comes naturally to most women' into a profession requiring training, the question of uniform had been a frequent subject of debate. Intended originally to protect the wearer against infection as well as disrespectful behaviour from patients, uniform soon became a means by which to express the hierarchy within the developing profession. Caps, belts and aprons were deliberately designed to make otherwise self-effacing women recognisable in terms of training, experience and rank. Even if the dress was not too comfortable and, particularly later on, the cap quite ineffective, nurses themselves valued them as part of their professional identity and as an expression of belonging. Detailed rules existed for the appropriate way of wearing uniform, identifying occasions when sleeves were to be worn either rolled up or down, the badge pinned on the right or left hand side, and a pin cushion hung from the belt underneath and not on top of the apron. [9] Uniform could therefore be displayed either as the garb of the untouchable ministering angels and as vocational costume, or as the uniform of a disciplined army of females executing the orders of medical men.

Having established uniform as a 'must' it came as a surprise, at least to the curator, to discover how difficult it was to obtain representative items. Possible explanations could be found in both the question of 'ownership' of uniform as well as that of their practical use. In municipal hospitals in Liverpool, nurses did not 'own' their uniforms, but had to return them when they left the service, when they would then either be reissued or put to other good use, often ending up as dusters or cleaning rags. When perusing minutes of the Port Sanitary and Hospitals Committee, which in 1930 was given control over twenty of Liverpool's former workhouse hospitals and other institutions, it transpired that in 1936 a 'Nurses' Uniforms Sub-Committee' was formed. This was chaired by Councillor Elizabeth (Bessie) Braddock, a formidable woman with a keen interest in health matters who did much to improve conditions for patients and hospital staff. The Sub-Committee was to review the situation of nurses' uniforms in the hospitals in its jurisdiction and to make recommendations on standardisation. This idea was met with opposition from the Matrons, but at a meeting of the Sub-Committee which they had been instructed to attend they were simply presented with the proposed standardised uniforms for almost all the grades of nurses and ancillary staff in the Corporation's employ - from deputy matrons to maids.[10] The minutes of the Sub-Committee, which functioned for just over a year, give detailed information about colour, fabric and design. When the

new uniforms were issued on 1st January 1937, all former
uniform was to be collected and disposed of - causing the loss of
what would now be desirable museum pieces. [11]

For the collection of material evidence to be used in the exhibition it proved invaluable to have nurses on the working party.
They were able to tap into a network of contacts which eventually
generated, on loan or as gifts, the objects and images we were
looking for. There appeared to be a pattern in the kind of objects
nurses keep as tokens of their working life. There are the badges,
such as the membership badge of the Royal College of Nursing;
the badge of the General Nursing Council for England and Wales
(the State Registered Nurse badge); hospital badges; the district
nursing badge designed by Mrs William Rathbone for Queen
Victoria's Jubilee Institute, and badges obtained for long or high
standards of service. They represent positive achievement and
distinction and are also small enough to be taken by their owners
even into retirement accommodation. Nurses also treasure their
certificates, probably for similar reasons. They are evidence of
hard-won qualifications, often worked for during precious off-
duty hours, and are items which require little space. Not
surprisingly, the exhibition boasted a good display of badges and
certificates connected with Liverpool hospitals.

A trawl for equipment of 'tools of the trade' brought in an
interesting but limited selection of objects, the nature of which
prompted further questions. Some had the character of gift items,
such as a thermometer in a 'fancy' holder or a handsome set of
medicine measures in a leather case, too nice for daily use. Was
one allowed to use these in the hospital? Several pin cushions
were collected, objects, it appeared, specifically connected with
the Liverpool Royal Infirmary.[12] Some pieces of equipment were
used specifically by nurses - a bandage winder, a sterilising drum,
a set of antiquated looking injection needles. It was not always
clear how these came to be in nurses' personal possession, but
that question is of less interest than that of the near total
disappearance of this type of object from the hospitals. Clearly,
items of obsolete nursing equipment were quickly disposed of,

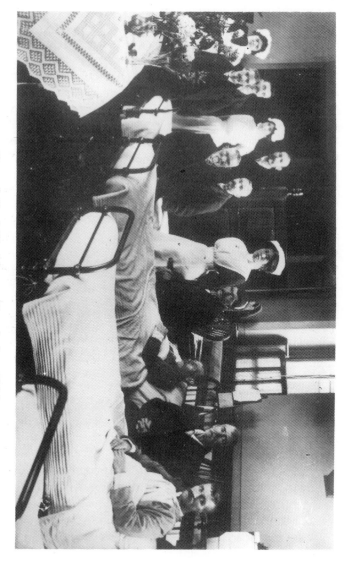

Toxteth Park Workhouse Hospital, c. 1914.

unlike instruments used by medical men which seem more frequently to end up in collections.

The search for images suitable for the exhibition was more successful and suggested, very tentatively, several identifiable categories. The earlier photographs, from about 1880 to 1914, mainly in public collections (The University of Liverpool and Liverpool Record Office), seem to have been taken mainly by professional photographers. They are almost invariably static and posed, and can be further subdivided. The first subgroup shows large wards with polished floors, a single table or desk in the middle (the ward sister's ?) with flowers or pot plants on top, rows of beds against the walls, with or without patients peeping from underneath immaculate counterpanes, clearly instructed not to move a muscle. Demure but elegant looking nurses in mutton- sleeved uniforms stand dotted between the beds or surround the occasional medical man. Of course there are exceptions to this format, such as a rather endearing photograph of nurses and male patients in the ward of the Toxteth Park Workhouse (now Sefton General Hospital) dating from around 1914. Also a posed picture, it seems to have been taken with the aim of showing people rather than the hospital environment and was perhaps meant to be sent home to family and relatives. Would it be significant that the latter was taken in a low status Poor Law Hospital as opposed to the prestigious Royal Infirmary? The second subgroup is equally formal. It is the year photograph either of a hospital's entire nursing staff, grouped in a bright white pyramid with a few darker clad dignitaries in the centre, or a smaller group of stiffly arranged nurses from a specific ward or training group. A delightful exception to this is a photograph which was lent by a member of the public and dates from 1908, showing nurses from Fazakerley Hospital at a fancy dress ball.

Images of nurses actually at work, nursing, seem to be rare before the 1930s. This may well be due to the limitations of photographic technology but perhaps also to restrictions on the use of the camera inside hospitals. One can speculate whether photographs taken during that earlier period were intended mainly to

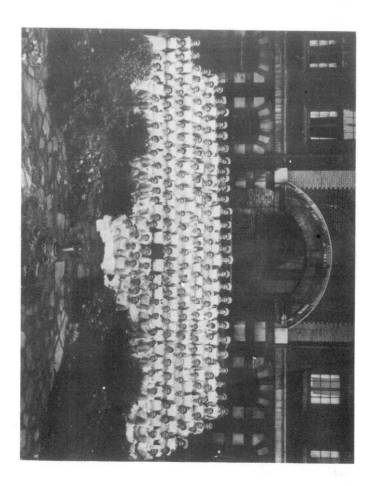

Nursing staff of the Liverpool Royal Infirmary, early 1950s

reinforce the carefully constructed public image of nurses: unobtrusive, serving, disciplined, capable.

Photographs in private possession and of a later date present a different category - individual snapshots and even whole albums with material which reveal more of the social side of nursing life. Nurses around a piano, rehearsing for Christmas carolling; taking part in inter-hospital tennis tournaments, or simply fooling around off-duty. These pictures show the non-stereotypical side of nurses: young women capable of enjoying life and taking part in a range of activities. There also surfaced some photographs of work situations taken by amateurs - a series of pictures in the operating theatre of the Royal Infirmary; nurses from the Children's Hospital cuddling their young patients or a midwife holding a baby surrounded by a beaming family group. No doubt the availability of such informal photographs has something to do with the popularisation of the use of cameras, but perhaps also with a more relaxed view of what nurses ought to be like.

The display which eventually was put together was, judging by comments in the visitors' book, well-received. The night of the Private View attracted large numbers of retired nurses as well as nurses currently working in Liverpool hospitals, and developed into an event resembling a reunion. There was no question that seeing the nursing profession celebrated in a museum gratified many visitors. Despite the positive way in which the exhibition had been received, the curator of the exhibition could not help feeling somewhat dissatisfied with the end product. This was partly because so much had been left out, not just because there was too little space but also because aspects of nursing life had deliberately been left unexplored. The curator's initial ignorance of nursing matters had been an asset insofar as it encouraged the nurses on the working party to consider aspects of their work which they had taken for granted as possibly open to different interpretation. Being of a similar age group and having training and worked in the same hospital they held similar ideas about what makes good nursing practice and about the profession in general. A broader-based working party, representative of the experience of nurses who had trained and worked in Liverpool's

Nurses of the Liverpool Maternity Hospital, Oxford Road, c. 1938.

other, that is, municipal (ex-workhouse) hospitals, might well have revealed different views and attitudes and given a different shape or direction to the exhibition project. Something of this was glimpsed when, during the research period, the curator interviewed a small number of nurses who had worked in the workhouse hospitals as well as two district nurses with experience of midwifery. Too small a sample to be representative or to allow for firm conclusions, it confirmed the feeling that there was much still to be explored about local nursing, such as possible links between class background, schooling, choice of hospital, further training and career opportunity. Talking about career choice, several interviewees recalled that careers advisers, such as they were at the time, would direct girls with an aspiration for nursing towards different Liverpool hospitals depending on school and family background. Generally speaking secondary modern school girls were assumed to be material for municipal hospitals whilst grammar school girls, having at first been counselled against choosing nursing as a career, were advised to apply to a teaching hospital. Irish girls were more likely to end up in a municipal hospital than Scottish and Welsh girls, who had no problems finding posts in the Liverpool Royal Infirmary. No clear reasons were given for this or, if they were, were vaguely ascribed to custom.

There was also the effect of marriage on a career. How were married nurses viewed by their single colleagues, especially their superiors, and more specifically in different hospitals with different staffing pressures? Linked to this was the level of control over nurses' social life inside and outside the confines of the hospital setting and exercised through the hierarchy headed by an all-powerful matron. One interviewee was prepared to discuss in some detail issues such as working conditions and pay, as she had been involved with early attempts to organise nurses into a trade union. In a profession, however, where members are caught between the pressure of high public esteem for unselfish caring and the need simply to make a living, how were nurses who expressed sympathy towards trade unionisation viewed by their peers and superiors? Limited evidence seems to suggest that efforts to unionise were received more favourably by nurses in municipal than in voluntary hospitals, although more work needs to be done before any firm conclusions can be drawn. The nurses interviewed, although not refusing to talk about any of these matters, needed a good deal of encouragement to do so, almost as if they thought themselves to be disloyal or indiscreet and damaging the public image of the profession by doing so.

Even if more factual information of this nature had been available to the working party, it is difficult to see how it could have been translated into visual displays. The few interviews undertaken did illustrate, however, the danger of relying exclusively on literary and material evidence as this can easily lead to an interpretation which is altogether too uncritical, or 'starry eyed'. 'This exhibition doesn't show at all what it was really like', at least one visitor (a retired nurse) snapped to the curator on the night of the Private View.

With the aim that nurses' own experiences should be central, perhaps the work should have started with interviews - oral history - instead of library research. Perhaps the exhibition would have benefitted from a primarily thematic approach (for example, exploring issues like recruitment, training, social life, hospital hierarchy) instead of fitting themes into a chronology, as the exhibition did. Even so, to find objects and images illustrating the themes would have been just as problematic.

In the event, the collaboration between museum staff and members of the public (the working party) did not end with the exhibition. Precisely because of the group's realisation of the limitations of available literary and material evidence, and the conviction that more research and better access to existing sources was necessary, the working group set itself three further objectives. The first one was to establish an oral history project. With the assistance of generous grants made by the Eleanor Rathbone Charitable Trust, the Liverpool Royal Infirmary Training School Nurses' League, Liverpool Health Authority (Trust Funds), and South Sefton (Merseyside) Health Authority (Trust Funds) a pilot project was launched in August 1991. Over the succeeding eighteen months, Mrs Frances Trees, as part-time

Research Assistant, completed a number of interviews with former nurses who had trained and/or worked in Liverpool. The success of this project has led to a generous grant from the Wellcome Trust to enable a major oral history project to be launched, covering the history of nursing on Merseyside.

The second objective was the listing of sources in such a way as to make them more accessible for research into local nursing history. This work was undertaken by the Assistant Archivist of the University of Liverpool and is now available to would-be researchers and interested members of the public. [13]

The third objective was to publish a volume of essays on local nursing history based mainly on personal reminiscences. It was hoped that such a volume would not only illustrate the value of oral history work but also encourage more research into local nursing history generally. The result of this work lies before you.

Notes

[1] Maggie Andrews (ed.), *Who Cared before the NHS? A Photographic Exhibition of the Development of Health and Welfare Services in the Mersey Region* (Liverpool, [1986])

[2] The collection and exhibition policy of the Merseyside Museum of Labour History was restricted to regional history.

[3] See above, p.1. For Liverpool, some information can be found in publications dealing with the history of individual hospitals.

[4] Gwen Hardy, *William Rathbone and the Early History of District Nursing* (Ormskirk, 1981)

[5] Ibid.

[6] See below, ch.9.

[7] Some work has been done by the late Gwen Hardy on the analysis of a private register of probationer nurses, covering the period 1862-88, until recently thought to be the only such surviving register for the period. Since then the official register covering the period, and comprising three volumes, has been identified in Liverpool Record Office.

[8] A similar problem faced John Adams, a nurse teacher in Kettering, who has collected over a hundred obsolete devices connected with nursing. See Daloni Carlisle, 'The History Man', Nursing Times, 23 September 1992, pp.38-39.

[9] See below, p.56

[10] Minutes of the Nurses' Uniforms Sub-Committee of the Port Sanitary and Hospitals Committee. Liverpool Record Office, 352 MIN/HOS 12/1.

[11] Minute no.3 of 3 September 1936 reads: 'All uniform dress, belts, collars, cuffs, coats, capes and caps (with the exception of Army caps and 4" stiff cuffs - which will still be worn by Sisters - also the aprons which may be easily altered to the new style) be transferred to one Centre, either to be disposed of or made into useful items such as butchers' aprons, etc; also that existing capes be altered for use as children's dressing gowns'.

[12] See below, p.56

[13] See below, ch.9. As noted, copies of a more extensive list of sources may be purchased upon application to Mr Allan at the University of Liverpool Archives.

Chapter 3
On the District
Winifred Froom

'DISTRICT NURSE'. So the disc on the car informed me, and as I passed she came down the garden path in her smart uniform and jaunty pill-box hat. Inevitably my thoughts return to the time when I, too, was a district nurse, or 'on the district', as we used to say. No smart car for us, we covered the miles on a bicycle. Some of the others went in for dropped handlebars, quite an innovation in those days, but I trusted to an old-fashioned Raleigh, the 'sit-up-and-beg' kind. On the carrier was strapped my black bag, containing a few dressings, forceps and an enema syringe. That was about all. In front of me was my bicycle basket, into which all kinds of articles found their way: a posy of flowers from some patient's garden, even my hat, which was discarded whenever possible.

I trained as a district nurse in Liverpool in 1946, by which time I had experienced different sorts of nursing and had worked in a number of Liverpool hospitals. From 1938 to 1941 I had been a probationer and gained my S.R.N at Mill Road, then a 600-bed municipal hospital; worked for a year as a staff nurse at Broadgreen; done six months midwifery training at Smithdown Road Hospital; trained for two years in ophthalmic nursing at St Paul's Eye Hospital and a year in the Venereal Diseases Clinic at Mill Road (always referred to as the Special Clinic). But of all the branches of nursing I studied, district work was the most satisfying. In it we met the patients in their own environment. In hospital beds they always reminded me of dolls in boxes, tightly tucked in. In their own homes they were people as well as patients, and the district nurse almost became a member of the family, not just somebody in authority. Of course, we exercised some influence and were appealed to for advice and assistance. And we were trusted with the front door key's hiding-place too.

Our uniform dresses were delphinium blue and over them we wore starched white aprons. As we moved from one patient's

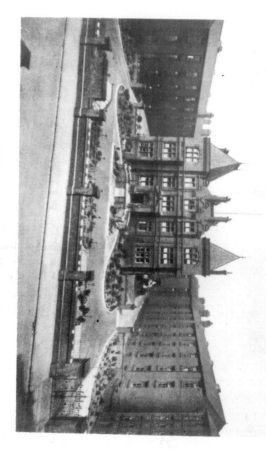

Mill Road Infirmary, c. 1939.

home to the next, the corners of these were carefully folded in and pinned at the waist so that the front of the apron did not come into contact with our coats. Our coats were of gaberdine and we wore little hats, like deerstalkers.

Every working day started at 8.30 a.m. when we assembled in the duty room of the Nurses' Home and were given our lists of patients for the morning. It was customary to visit new patients and diabetics first, the former to be informed of what to prepare for the nurse's visit, the latter to receive their injection of insulin, so that they could get on with their breakfast! In such cases the patients were responsible for making sure everything was ready for the nurse's arrival: the syringe and needle, surgical spirit and cotton wool swab and insulin would all be put out in a dish so that the nurse could draw up and give the injection quickly and get on with her rounds, and the patient enjoy the first meal of the day. So that the instruments were as sterile as possible, patients were given lists of instructions about how to get them ready for the nurse's visit, though we could never be sure that all our patients did exactly as they had been told. A normal household dish was used to hold the syringe and needles. Dish, syringe and needles would all be sterilised by boiling in a large pan on the patient's stove

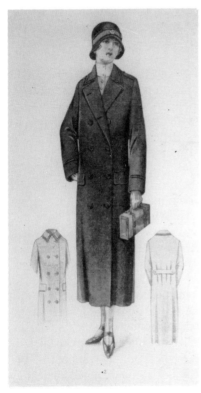

'New costume for District Nurses', as proposed in a pamphlet published by the General Nursing Council, 1937.

and sterile water obtained by boiling a kettle and storing the boiled water in a jar. Swabs, syringes and needles all came from the local chemist on production of a prescription from the patient's doctor.

Usually such visits took only a few minutes. Most patients were well aware of the procedure, but in the days when doctors and nurses were held in great awe, some diabetics had not dared to ask for their condition and its treatment to be explained. Nor did some understand why it was important for them to keep to their diets. One old lady I visited, whose arm was pitted with needle pricks, had never been told, and when I explained, as simply as possible, was astounded. 'Well, fancy that, nobody ever told me before, not even the doctor.'

One of my regular patients was an elderly woman who had suffered a stroke and was confined to bed. Happily, she lived with an affectionate and competent daughter, who was quite capable of nursing her mother, with the help of a daily visit from the district nurse. 'And father will be able to fetch and carry for us,' she told me on my first visit.

In the months that followed, the old woman and her husband proved to be a real Darby and Joan, the former only leaving his wife's side to retire discreetly while we attended to her needs. Much later I met the daughter and was told that the old lady had died, and I wasn't surprised to learn her husband had died a fortnight later. 'They existed for each other,' said their daughter.

District nurses were often given the task of checking and renewing dressings of patients who had been discharged from hospital after surgery, but whose wounds were not yet fully healed. In the case of post-operative dressings, it was only necessary to take off the old dressing and put on a new one. But this was before the days of the pre-sterilised and individually-wrapped dressings that we are now familiar with. Patients or their families had to provide them, and the nurse would give instructions for preparing them by baking squares of lint and gauze in a biscuit tin, in the oven! The cooled tin would be laid out ready for the nurse's visit, along with a supply of sterile water and surgical spirit.

32

Patients who had contracted such minor but unpleasant conditions as thread worms were also referred to the district nurses, both for treatment and for advice about preventing their recurrence. The parasites are easily spread from one person to another, especially where children are concerned, and it was important that the district nurse gave careful instructions about personal hygiene and the preparation of food.

Patients needing dressings and treatment for minor complaints did not stay long on the district nurse's visiting list. Others, though, needed care for a long time. As we visited regularly over weeks and months it was inevitable that we got to know the patients and their families intimately. In such cases, the nurse's role was to support the family and to help with any tasks that they were unable to perform. One of my patients, for instance, received a daily visit for the simple reason that her caring daughter hadn't the strength to wash her bed-ridden mother, who weighed at least twenty stones! This enormous lady reclined against a tower of pillows in a big double bed. We toiled together, the daughter and I, washing her, rolling her from side to side to change the bottom sheet, treating her pressure areas by rubbing with methylated spirit and dusting with talcum powder, and all the time she puffed and smiled in the most amiable fashion, her three chins wobbling like unset jellies, but never saying a word! Every day the routine was the same. Once we had finished and the patient, fresh and comfortable, relaxed on her pillows, her daughter disappeared to make a cup of tea for each of us. Caring for such patients is easier these days, with the provision of a laundry service and rubber sheeting and equipment like hoists and back-rests, but it is still hard and heavy work.

Sometimes on my list of bed-baths and dressings, there appeared an unusual task. On one occasion a local doctor had asked that the district nurse visit an old lady who could not cut her toenails. No wonder, for her bosom jutted out like a shelf and she could not see her feet. Nowadays she would perhaps attend the Health Centre and receive attention from the chiropodist, but before the establishment of the National Health Service this would not have been available, except privately.

Injections, dressings, bed-baths and treatments of minor ailments would occupy every morning. Once we had finished, we went back to the Nurses' Home in Brookside Avenue for lunch. Thirteen of us lived there, one of several such homes in the city, under the supervision of the Superintendent and her deputy. Living in a district nurses' home was quite different from being in residence in a hospital. The community was much smaller and life was less formal. We even addressed each other differently. In hospital we were usually called 'Nurse' by patients and colleagues alike; on the district we referred to each other as Miss, or, if we were particularly friendly, by our surnames! I don't remember ever calling my colleagues by their first name or hearing mine used. For many of us, used to the rigid discipline and petty regulations of hospital nursing, it came as a pleasant surprise to find ourselves treated as responsible trained nurses. We were even issued with our own personal latch key to use after an evening out. No longer did we have to ask for a late pass and explain where we going and when we expected to be back. In addition, we were allowed to entertain visitors from time to time, and there was a little sitting-room for the purpose, and facilities for making tea and providing refreshments. Our own rooms were very comfortable too, with individual electric fires, although we had to feed coins into the slot from our own pockets. The care of the home and the catering was the responsibility of a Superintendent, who supervised the cook and the cleaner.

Off-duty time was quite generous. We had one completely free day a week, and every afternoon off until 4.30 p.m., when we went out again to attend the patients who had to be treated more than once a day. But there were not many of them and we were invariably back again for our evening meal at 6.30 p.m. The hours that followed were our own. There was a rota in case somebody was needed for an emergency visit, but with thirteen of us on it, we did not have to be 'on call' very often. Sometimes being 'on call' could be a sad experience. Many of our patients were elderly and sometimes we were asked by the doctor to go to lay out someone who had died. I well remember such a visit. As I left the house after performing the last offices for his wife, her grieving husband gave me a present of two new-laid eggs from the hens he kept in the yard.

We spent our off-duty in various ways. Sometimes we made up a party to visit a cinema or theatre, but many preferred to stay in the sitting-room, knitting or reading. The conversation was general, and not a great deal of time was spent reviewing current affairs: for the most part, the nurses were only mildly interested in politics and were more intent on passing their examinations and becoming Queen's Nurses. Our Superintendent had broad interests, though, and always discouraged talking 'shop', especially at meal-times.

As well as practical work on the district, we attended lectures on public health and hygiene, social welfare and giving advice and assistance whenever possible. For these we joined nurses from other districts of the city at the headquarters of the Queen Victoria District Nursing Service in Princes Road. Our months of training sped past, and the day of the written examination came and went, to be followed by a practical demonstration of home nursing.

For this part of the examination we selected three or four of our cases, warning them beforehand that they were to be leading ladies or men in the coming event, so that they could have everything ready for the visit, when we would be accompanied by the examiner. I selected one of my regular patients, someone who needed to have bed-baths. This was not the large lady in the double bed, but a plucky little person whose limbs were so twisted with osteo-arthritis that she was quite helpless, except for an indomitable sense of humour. I also included someone who needed a dressing - a lady who suffered a severe scald of her leg, which was now healing nicely! At no time, however, did she allow this misfortune to interfere with her household duties if she could help it. She managed to do all kinds of jobs sitting down, like washing small garments in the kitchen sink, and one day I found her shelling peas into a bowl in her lap. So I was not surprised to find her sitting in her chair, with a bowl between her knees, mixing a cake when the examiner and I arrived. Unfortunately, we were unable to wait for it to be baked, otherwise a slice would have accompanied the inevitable cup of tea, which was made by her husband on her behalf. Few visits were not accompanied by the invitation to share a cuppa ... sometimes so

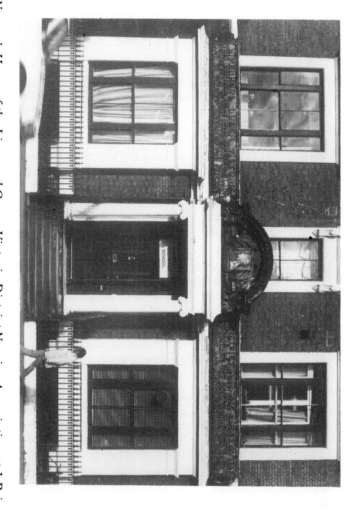

The Central Nurses' Home of the Liverpool Queen Victoria District Nursing Association at 1 Princes Road. The building is now used as a school.

many were offered that time was too short to accept them all. And on our rounds at Christmas, offers of tea were changed to offers of sherry, or port wine! Fortunately there was not much traffic on the roads because fewer people owned cars and petrol was still rationed; in fact the greatest hazard for the district nurse - especially if she had enjoyed some Christmas hospitality - was posed by the tram-lines which could grip a bicycle wheel fast and send its rider flying.

Two more cases completed my list, and then we returned to the Nurses' Home for lunch. In a very short time I learned that I had been successful and was presented with the open evidence of my success - two small shoulder tabs to be stitched to my gaberdine coat, and a certificate pronouncing me a Queen's Nurse. After that, my year of training was over, and I started my year of service with the District Nurses' Association, one of the conditions in my contract.

Once the National Health Service was established, district nurses were incorporated in it. This brought changes almost immediately. Increased equipment arrived at the nurses' homes, to be borrowed by people who needed it: things like rubber sheeting, back rests, crutches, and wheelchairs were made available for patients' use. Later on, a laundry service was promised, and sheets provided for people who needed frequent changes of bed-linen. Diabetic patients, if mobile, were encouraged to attend for their injections, if possible, or else taught to administer their own insulin at home. Inevitably some of the close contact between district nurse and patient suffered.

It is likely, however, that all these changes came about more slowly in country districts, where it was still more practical for the nurse to continue to visit patients in their homes, although even there some local authorities started to use ambulances, mini-ambulances and voluntary car drivers to transport patients to clinics and hospitals for injections, physiotherapy and day centres.

My training and experience was in the city. However, we were able to spend a few days on a country district as the guest of the resident district nurse, who was invariably a midwife too. It was altogether a delightful experience. I still remember mine. It was October, when the autumn tints were enriching the scenery in which I found myself. My hostess, the district nurse who was also the district midwife, met me at the little railway station in Shropshire and took me back to her cosy cottage, complete with roses round the door, chintz-covered chairs, and bone china crockery. The next morning we set off in her small car - a bicycle would have been quite inadequate to cover the miles between the cases she had to attend. In the homely parlours, or in the tiny bedrooms, we conducted much the same kind of work as on the city rounds; dressings, bed baths, and of course a maternity case. There was the same intimacy between nurse and patient, the same anticipation of our arrival, but the difference lay in the greater responsibility borne by the nurse, alone in her cottage, with only the telephone to link her with the doctor or the nearest hospital. Sometimes two nurses shared a district and a cottage and could help each other and organise their work so that each could have regular time off. Visiting a country district was a delightful experience but, lasting only three days, it wasn't possible to judge whether I could have coped with it for weeks, or months. So I returned to the city laden with apples and early chrysanthemums and a feeling that perhaps the city district was my place; the place where humble dwellings jostled with detached and semi-detached villas, where outside toilets contrasted with the indoor facilities of the latter - one house in a better type of district which we covered actually had a sunken bath! It was a long way away from the original idea of the District Nurses' Association 'to nurse the poor in their own homes'.

During my time as a district nurse, the prospect of a National Health Service being established before long was something that interested and affected all of us, and some of us watched developments keenly. When a meeting on the subject took place in a local hall, the Superintendent encouraged half a dozen nurses to go along. The meeting was organised by the Socialist Medical Association, of which I had been an active member for a long time. Membership of the S.M.A was acceptable to the nursing authorities, and I could not help but reflect on an earlier excursion into the political arena when I had been a pupil midwife. Becoming a pupil again, when some of us had held responsible hospital posts was quite difficult, but we were all prepared for that in order to gain an important qualification. We were even prepared for the drop in salary that the training entailed. But we were not prepared for the poor working conditions and inadequate off-duty. Twenty-two of us had the temerity to join a trade union and we reaped the disapproval of the authorities; membership of the appropriate trade union was not encouraged until some years later. Probably the entry into nursing of many members of the Army Medical Corps, demobilised after the end of the Second World War, coupled with the introduction of the National Health Service, helped to accelerate union membership.

However, my immediate future had to be decided and for a while I wondered about continuing with district work, but ultimately decided to return to ophthalmic nursing, which I found nearly as satisfying as district nursing!

The new Health Service was already a reality; just an infant service, it is true, but with the right upbringing it had the possibility of growing into a healthy adult. No more flag days, nor street collections; no more voluntary helpers. Or so we thought. But I like to think there will always be a role for the district nurse to play, acting as go-between between patient and hospital.

Chapter 4
Other People's Children
Gwynneth Rowe

The Liverpool Infirmary for Children was the first children's
hospital in Britain. It was opened for the treatment of out-patients
in 1851, a year before the famous Hospital for Sick Children at
Great Ormond Street in London, and was later to be known as The
Royal Liverpool Children's Hospital. Its first buildings were in
Upper Hill Street, and before the move to the purpose-built
hospital in Myrtle Street, whose foundation stone was laid in
1866, it had occupied premises successively in Great George
Street and Hope Street. Alterations and additions have been
made to the original buildings in Myrtle Street, principally since
the hospital was taken over by the National Health Service in
1948, but the nucleus of those early ones still stands.

A further development in the care of sick children in the city came
with the foundation of the Liverpool Country Hospital for
Chronic Diseases of Children. It opened in temporary premises
at West Kirby on the Wirral in 1899 and moved into a purpose-
built hospital on a site overlooking the River Dee at Heswall in
1909. The hospital was granted the title of The Royal Liverpool
Country Hospital for Children in 1910. And in 1917 Thingwall
Hall, Barnston was acquired and used as a Recovery Hospital.
The ee branches together contained 400 beds for children from
birth to the age of sixteen years.

The nursing of sick children demands special skills and in the
early years of the twentieth century a course was devised which
was designed to develop them. The Supplementary Register for
Sick Children's Nurses was separate from State Registration, and
candidates were allowed to start the three-year training for
membership of the Register at the age of seventeen-and-a-half
years. Students who continued with a general nurse training on
qualifying experienced a certain amount of repetition and it was

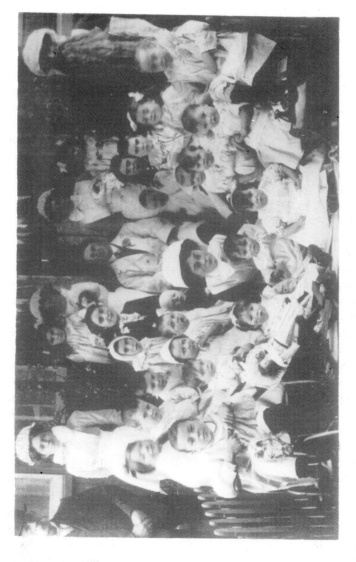

Children, nursing staff and a doctor at the Liverpool Infirmary for Children, Myrtle Street, c. 1910.

to avoid this that the combined S.R.N./R.S.C.N. scheme was developed.

When the author started her training in March 1937, the training of probationers, the term used before the currently familiar one of student nurses, was haphazard, as recruits were accepted in ones or twos, with no provision for any preliminary training before being sent to work on the wards. Each was told to equip herself with a watch with a second hand and a pair of dressing scissors, and to report to the hospital at a certain time on a certain day, dressed in a uniform made to measure by the firm of Andrew Brown, in Paradise Street, Liverpool. By 5.30 p.m. the new recruit had said good-bye to her escort, more often than not one of her parents, had nervously drunk a cup of tea, and, wearing a Sister Dora cap, blue and white striped uniform with a stiff collar, and rigid white starched belt and cuffs, had been delivered to a ward as a new member of staff to work until 8.00 p.m.

It was a daunting experience. There was a new vocabulary to be learned, and a rigid discipline to get used to. Sister's instructions had to be followed without questioning. Sometimes this led to amusing misunderstandings. Abbreviations were not often used, but on one occasion a ward sister requested a probationer of a few days' experience to go to the basement and collect a T.C.I. (An abbreviation for To Come In - meaning a new patient for admission.) The probationer was too afraid to admit that she did not know the meaning of the abbreviation, and was unable to find anyone in the basement who might have been able to explain it to her. Mystified, but fearful to return to the ward empty-handed, she noticed a large china jug in the corner and walked back to the ward with the article in her hand. The busy ward sister was not amused, but did acknowledge that the probationer had used her initiative!

After the first six months of training, probationers experienced their first taste of night-duty, generally for a three-month period with two free nights off a month. This was an exciting novelty for some nurses, who enjoyed the idea of staying awake and active all night; but for others, especially those who found it

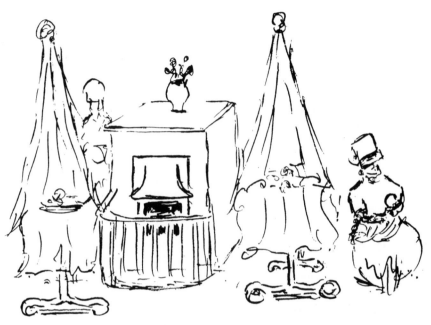

Swing cots, The Royal Liverpool Children's Hospital, c.1940.

impossible to sleep properly during the day, it was an exhausting and difficult time. Night nurses slept on the top floor of the Nurses' Home, and all other nurses living there were careful to keep noise to a minimum during the day. But nothing could stop the street noises and the bells of the nearby cathedral disturbing the sleep of the night nurses. The problems of tiredness were compounded when probationers on night duty were expected to attend lectures during the day, even though they had been working all the previous night.

The night started at 8.00 p.m., when night sister reported to Matron to hear about activities in the hospital during the day and the night-nurses went to their wards to receive a full report on the health of the children on the ward and instructions about the care they were to have for the next twelve hours. It ended at 8.00 a.m. the following day. It was usual for two nurses to be allocated to each ward, and an extra nurse - known as a 'runner' - to have responsibility for relieving staff for meals and for giving extra help as and when required. Although many of the children could be expected to sleep for several hours, there were many occasions when the ward was as busy at night as it had been during the day. Routine tasks, like recording the temperature, pulse and respiration of the patients, were performed at set times; tiny babies fed at regular intervals; urine tested for abnormalities; used nappies sluiced; fluid charts, recording the intake and output of individual children, filled in and totalled; temperature and admission books ruled and the unpredictable needs of sick children met.

Like their colleagues on day duty, night nurses had to be prepared for the death of some of their small patients. Few ever got used to it. Night sister was responsible for making sure that the child's parents were informed, perhaps by requesting the police to ask the parents to telephone the hospital, while the nurses, often tearfully, washed the body and wrapped it in a shroud ready to be taken to the hospital mortuary. This was a detached building in the back courtyard of the hospital. The bodies of older children had to be taken there on a mortuary trolley, but those of babies and young children could be taken in the arms of one of the nurses who had looked after them, often wrapped in a grey blanket in an attempt to disguise the nature of the bundle. This was always a painful experience for the nurses, and sometimes the journey across the courtyard had to be made two or three times during the night. On top of all this, the two nurses had to cope with unexpected emergency admissions.

Night sister did a round of all the wards in turn between 10.00 p.m. and 11.00 p.m., and woe betide the nurse who was unable to escort her round the ward and tell her the name, diagnosis and treatment of every child. Sometimes sister appeared when she was not expected and discovered high-spirited nurses engaging in less than professional activities. An example of the sort of behaviour that might occur was the occasion when a probationer kept herself awake on a night when the ward was quiet by decorating a child's straw hat, putting it on her head and then covering her arms with the long socks worn to the operating theatre by children about to have surgery. Pleased with the effect, she crept into the ward prepared to frighten her senior, who was writing the night report. But this was one of the times when night sister had decided to pay a surprise call; she was not amused to be greeted by such an apparition!

Night sister was not alone in her practice of making unexpected visits: in the days when Matron lived on the premises, she, too, might appear at any time of day or night to 'see how things were going'.

As well as helping out on the wards, the 'runner' on night-duty had to be prepared to turn her hand to a variety of tasks. While the hospital telephonist took her meal break, the 'runner' had to cope with the eccentricities of the hospital telephone exchange and to be responsible for connecting both internal and external calls. And she had to cook the night sister's meal and have it ready to be served promptly at 11.30 p.m. Night sisters experienced different degrees of culinary skill. Some, unwittingly, ate food which had suffered accidents. One summer evening the kitchen window had been left open, and the author, that night's 'runner', arrived to see a cat disappearing through the window with sister's supper, a lamb chop, in its mouth. Undaunted, the probationer

"Other Peoples Babies."

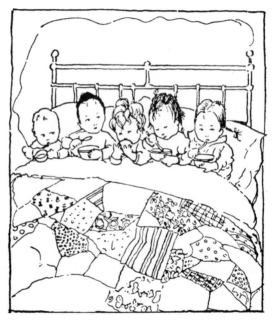

Greetings from *Gwynneth*

The Royal Liverpool Children's Hospital,

Myrtle Street.

Liverpool.

Greetings card from The Royal Liverpool Children's Hospital, c. 1938.

leapt through the lower window and retrieved the chop, which she washed and cooked and served to the sister, who was not told what had happened - nor, so far as is known, did she suffer any ill effects!

However busy she was, and whatever the needs of the nurses on the wards, the 'runner' was responsible for waking the twenty or so maids who slept in an upper dormitory alongside the hospital kitchen. One hearty knock on each door was all that there was time for - any maid who slept on had to rely on her friends to make sure she got to work on time: the nurse was far too busy to check that the sleepers had woken. Having done that, she had to go to the hospital kitchen and light the gas under the pans containing the patients' breakfast porridge.

Although both interesting and exhausting, night duty did not last for ever. Life on day duty also had its routines. One event viewed with some anxiety by the nurses was the annual spring clean. The patients were transferred to other wards while theirs was being turned out, and a nucleus of staff was left to assist the ward sister in scrubbing and cleaning. The terrazzo floor was thoroughly scrubbed by the ward maid, but the cleaning of the window sills and disinfecting of the walls was the nurses' job. At the same time equipment and instruments were checked and replaced, and missing objects searched for. When everything had been counted, cleaned and made ready for the next year's use, it was laid out for inspection, and sister escorted Matron while she checked the equipment against the inventory she kept in her office. Most missing articles were replaced from the hospital store by others of identical size and pattern, but thermometers had to be replaced by the nurses who had broken them, at the cost of one shilling (5p) for a clinical thermometer and three shillings (15p) for a lotion thermometer. (When a first-year probationer's salary in 1940 was £17 a year, this represented a large amount of money, especially if any nurse had been unfortunate enough to drop a whole container of thermometers!) At last all the ward equipment was replaced, and for one day all was correct, before articles began to disappear again to make the omissions for the following year!

At the same time as the ward was being cleaned, mattresses were sent to the bedding store to be re-covered as necessary. This was the responsibility of the store-room staff. Not so the pillows. Making them ready for another year's wear and tear was the nurses' job, and an unpopular one it was! The insides of new pillow covers were prepared by being rubbed with hard soap, so that the feathers once replaced would not work their way through the covers. Once this was done, new feathers were stuffed into the covers which were then sewn up. The nurses given this task always ended up with feathers all over their uniform, up their noses and in their hair.

Nursing made great demands on the health of those young women who worked very long hours, often in difficult conditions, and the physical care of the probationer left much to be desired. Frequently nurses' complaints received little sympathy and any who took time off because they were sick had to cope with the knowledge that they were making extra work for their colleagues, especially on night duty, when staffing was very tight. Ailments such as septic fingers, boils and jaundice were more common in the 1940s than the 1990s and those suffering from them were often forced to cope with their symptoms in silence. There was, however, an administrative system for dealing with illness. Sick probationers had to report to home sister in a morning clinic, and any needing dressings or poultices in the evening were sent to see theatre sister in the anaesthetic room next to the operating theatre. But the system did not always work well. The present writer who, in 1938, was certain that the stomach pains she was suffering were due to appendicitis, and said so, received short shrift from home sister because 'no nurse ever diagnosed herself'. In desperation she sought help from the Matron, who did take her seriously, and she was in the operating theatre at Myrtle Street within hours for an appendicectomy.

Although it was unsystematic, training was important and provision was made for probationers to attend lectures by doctors and senior nurses. Attendance at these lectures was compulsory, usually during the nurse's off-duty hours, or before or after a spell of night-duty. Examinations had to be passed and the timing of these, too, failed to take into account the pressures experienced by tired nurses, some of whom had been working on the wards all the previous night.

Overall responsibility for nurse-training lay with the sister tutors, usually helpful and anxious to make themselves available to the nurses in their care, but often frustrated in their work because of the extra demands made on their time. For example, it was not unusual for them to be required to supervise probationers' meals in the dining-room, or to have to work in the administrative office in the evening on top of their teaching duties. The supervision of meals was normally performed by the Matron, or her assistant, and they used these times to comment on disciplinary matters, such as the tidiness and cleanliness of the probationers' uniforms. Meal-times were also the occasion for the publication of examination results and 'change lists' - that is, the re-allocation to wards, drawn up by the Matron. Nurses attending the dining-room for a meal were expected to wear either full uniform, complete with cap, or to be in mufti.

The work done by nurses in Liverpool was recognised in a very practical way by a generous benefactor. The Walter Harding Fund for Nurses provided a ticket for a day's excursion to Llandudno, with time to walk round the Great Orme, or alternatively a visit to the Playhouse Theatre in Liverpool. As the numbers of staff grew this became too difficult to administer, and the money was used instead to contribute to a Christmas party in the hospital.

(Another example of Mr Harding's generosity was his gift to the hospital in 1935 of a collection of valuable nineteenth-century French toys. In 1974 the Board of Governors agreed that these should be sold at Sotheby's to raise funds for both Myrtle Street and Heswall. The most exciting toy in the collection was a crocodile, nearly three feet long, and accurate in every detail. Its legs and mouth moved, the latter to show a set of sharp pointed teeth. This was auctioned for £300, the highest sum paid for any of the toys. A figure of a mandolin player in a white silk waistcoat with lace trimmings, which moved in time to music, raised £230.

A monkey, which rose from within a papier-mache pineapple, realised £160, which was £10 more than an appealing white fluffy rabbit, whose ears rose as it moved from within a cabbage. Altogether the auction made £1,634.)

Little emphasis was given to teaching probationers about the emotional needs of young children, and much ward routine was directed towards cleanliness and efficiency and obedience to the doctors' demands, often at the expense of psychological support of the child, ill and away from home. A rigid ward routine, which insisted that meals were served punctually and that tasks such as bathing, toileting and bedmaking all had to be done at certain times, left little space for comforting the unhappy child or playing with the bored one. When doctors did their ward rounds, small patients were expected to maintain absolute silence and to remain still in tidy beds whose counterpanes were pulled straight and corners neatly mitred. Children in The Royal Liverpool Children's Hospital even wore a sort of uniform. During the day they were dressed in pink day coats which had been beautifully feather-stitched by the ladies of the Linen League, and after 5.30 p.m., when the blinds had been lowered - probably by the most junior probationer - fawn night-coats were worn.

In order to allow for doctors' and Matron's rounds and necessary medical procedures, specifically nursing tasks had to be timetabled into the hour or so before and after the children had eaten their lunch. This was the point in the day when nurses combed the children's hair with fine-toothed combs and treated those unlucky enough to have contracted head-lice. Treatment consisted of covering the infected scalp with oil of sassafras, obtained from the bark of a North American tree, and covering it with a piece of old linen. The whole was then covered with an intricate scalp bandage known as a capelline, a work of art made with two-inch gauze roller bandages applied in an intricate criss-cross pattern, and left in position until the next day. Other lunch-hour tasks included rinsing large quantities of used nappies in the sluice room, before counting them and putting them in large linen bags and sending them to the hospital laundry. The children's lockers were also cleaned regularly, their brushes and combs washed and clean clothes given out. From lunch-time onwards large wooden containers on wheels would appear in the corridor outside the ward. These contained clean ward linen - sheets, draw-sheets, pillow cases, towels and nappies, as well as children's clothing. One of the probationers would be given the job of checking all the laundry against the list sent with the dirty linen and then replacing clean stock tidily in the linen cupboard.

The wooden 'changing trolley' was used for an important nursing procedure which took place every four hours, and was not performed just during the lunch-hour. Nappies were changed and care taken to see that all the children were dry and comfortable. Stored in the sluice, the trolley was equipped with a basin, a bucket, soap, flannels, clean sheets and nappies and a 'back tray' containing castor oil and zinc-oxide cream for soothing the sore buttocks of babies and young children confined to bed.

Visiting was discouraged, except for babies and those children who were dangerously ill, and the author remembers children, crying with homesickness, waving to their parents from the balcony or window. Families and friends who wanted to leave gifts for the children had to hand them at a specified time to the sister or staff nurse, who met them in the basement, well away from the ward, and often returned laden with sweets, biscuits and lollipops. These were shared among all the children well enough to eat them, and a sweet round often took place after the midday medicine round. But there were aspects of the children's wards which may have helped to alleviate feelings of homesickness; coal fires, surrounded by a large iron fireguard, supplemented the central heating and the flickering light must have given a comforting glow at night. The most seriously ill babies were nursed in treasure cots - swing cots with delicate voile coverings, made by the ladies of the Linen League - on either side of the fireplace, and it was a matter of prestige amongst the nurses as to who undertook the role of caring for their occupants. It was the staff nurses' task to wash and starch the coverings in the ward kitchen when necessary.

The children had few highlights to cheer their lives, but during November administrators from the Town Hall used to 'phone to let the hospital know when the Lord Mayor's State Coach would be passing and would arrange for it to pause outside the hospital so that as many children as possible could see it.

Christmas was always a mixture of happiness and sadness, as some children were too ill to appreciate what was going on, but the ward staff went to great lengths to make sure that there was lots to enjoy for those who were less seriously sick. The wards were made festive with decorations and suitable pictures painted on the windows by talented - and sometimes not-so-talented - nurses. And every ward boasted a Christmas tree. Father Christmas's arrival on Christmas Eve was awaited with glee and excitement. The part of Father Christmas was usually taken by a junior doctor, who toured the wards between 10.00 p.m. and 11.00 p.m. at night, carrying a sack of presents. Needless to say, some children managed to stay awake to see him and his helpers fill the long, hospital-issue operation socks hung on the ends of their beds! Every child was given a present from the ward staff, and extra gifts were provided by various charities as well as local churches and schools, and even parents grateful for the ·care offered to their children. Boxing Day was known as Tree Day and the hospital was open from 2.00 p.m. to 4.30 p.m. for Friends of the Hospital. Sometimes, parents of the nurses visited and observed their daughters in action, and probably saw them in uniform for the first time.

Schooling was often neglected while the child was in hospital. But the Royal Liverpool Children's Hospital at Heswall was one of the first in the country to enjoy the added facility of a hospital school which, although it had the support of the local authorities, was not controlled by them. From as early as 1899 teachers, many of whom gave their services voluntarily, tried to make sure that the young patients had some formal education, and later a fully-qualified head-teacher was appointed. In 1960, children in the Liverpool hospital were included in the school.

Before antibiotics made the treatment of infection quicker and more certain, ward procedures were sometimes directed to reducing the effects of offensive wounds; in the orthopaedic wards, patients whose wounds smelled unpleasantly were aired off on the open balconies, muffled in woollies in the winter, and encouraged to watch the trams go by! And many treatments were aimed as much at relieving the symptoms of serious disease as attacking their cause. Medical wards frequently housed children with rheumatism and renal disorders, who were prescribed complete rest and nursed in so-called 'blanket beds'. Many children disliked this treatment, which meant that they were forced to lie between woollen blankets, were allowed only one pillow and were discouraged from making any movement.

Children with croup or other respiratory complaints were often nursed in steam tents. To make one of these, nurses removed the curtains from one of the screens normally used to surround a bed when treatment was being carried out and covered it with a sheet so that it made a sort of tent. This was positioned over the child's bed and inside it a boiling kettle was placed on a stand, so that the patient breathed warm, moist air. It may have helped them to breathe, but many children found the experience of lying under a semi-saturated sheet unpleasant.

Gastroenteritis was commonly found among children who lived in the sub-standard houses in the area around the hospital, and babies who caught it often became very dehydrated and had to be subjected to repeated and painful injections of saline just under the skin of the groin or under the arm.

Patients admitted to the Children's Hospital often came from poor families and were chronically under-nourished. For them convalescence was a vital part of the recovery process. Once the acute phase of their illness had been treated, such children were transported either to Thingwall Hall, Barnston, or the Royal Liverpool Children's Hospital at Heswall, in the hospital ambulances. The driver of the ambulance was the children's friend, and secreted packets of sweets for distraught passengers. Many of the children had never seen cows or other farm animals, so the 'country route' was frequently chosen, to allow them to enjoy the sights and sounds of the countryside.

Not all children who attended the hospital had to be admitted to one of the wards. The Casualty Department, situated in the basement of the hospital, gave prompt treatment to many babies and children brought there by a parent or an older brother or sister. The poverty of parts of inner-city Liverpool in the inter-war period meant that many such children were poorly clothed - some might even have been stitched into vests of brown paper - but in the Casualty Department they were assured of the best treatment available.

The separation of patients needing different types of specialist surgical treatment is a recent development, and in the 1940s all those children who needed surgery were admitted into general surgical wards. Some stayed only a short time. During the period when the removal of tonsils and adenoids was deemed to be desirable, many children were submitted to the 'guillotine' procedure and, so long as they did not bleed badly, were sent home at the end of the day.

Progress has been made with time and experience. On the one hand treatments have become more heroic. Electronic monitoring has replaced some of the nurses' observations and the elaborate tray and trolley settings for ward and theatre procedures have been replaced by disposable packs and a throw-away technique. Visiting is more relaxed, with parents more involved in their children's care and, thanks to antibiotics, the treatment of many children's illnesses has been simplified.

At the heart of the matter, a children's hospital is geared to the needs of infants and children from infancy until they leave school. The staff at Myrtle Street were always proud that any children coming to the desk at the hospital entrance, even without an adult in charge, would be taken seriously because it was their hospital.

Chapter 5

Christmas in Hospital

Mavis Gray

Whatever else be lost among the years,
Let us keep Christmas -
its meaning never ends;
Whatever doubts assail us, or what fears,
Let us hold close this day -
remembering friends!

Many families have special ways of celebrating Christmas and
pass on traditions from generation to generation, and the Liverpool Royal Infirmary family was no exception. Customs were
passed from one set of nurses to the next, so that although few can
now be certain when they started most can remember the important part that they played in the celebration of Christmas in
hospital. This account is based on the author's experiences
between 1951 and 1962, and includes memories supplied by
many of the nurses with whom she worked at the Liverpool Royal
Infirmary.

Often one of ward sister's most tiresome responsibilities, the
preparation of the off-duty rota, presented no problems over
Christmas. All the nursing staff, from Matron down to the most
junior probationers (known as 'pros') spent the entire day on
duty, and would have been disappointed had this not been the
case. Nearly all nursing staff lived in hospital accommodation
- residence was compulsory for probationers and charge nurses,
and encouraged for ward sisters - and the hospital community
expected to celebrate together. For many of them Christmas was
the high spot of the year.

But if the nursing staff expected to spend Christmas in hospital,
most of their patients did not: for many of them admission to
hospital was an unwelcome intrusion in their lives. But patients
and nurses shared at least one thing in common; they were
separated from their families, and the surrogate family was to be
found within the hospital.

Preparations for Christmas started, surreptitiously, well in advance, just in case the hospital was so busy in December that there was not enough time to fit them all in. The ward or departmental sister planned the design of the pin-cushions she would make and present to each member of her staff on Christmas morning. Yes, pin-cushions! It is not known when this practice started, but Miss Margaret Haynes recollects that the pin-cushions were in vogue when she was training in 1925 and it would appear that some of the sisters are wearing them in a photograph published in the booklet compiled by Betty Hoare (née Eaglesfield) and Beryl Phillips to commemorate the Centenary of the Training School.[1]

The pin-cushion each nurse at the Liverpool Royal Infirmary could expect to receive on Christmas morning would be equipped with a needle or two, straight pins, and safety pins (gold and stainless steel) and attached to a length of cord so that it could be worn either chatelaine fashion or pinned to the dress pocket underneath the apron. Designs of pin-cushions were numerous, influenced undoubtedly by the imagination and craft skills of the maker, not to mention the availability of suitable materials. Simple needle cases, some intricately decorated, competed for originality with cushions fashioned like bells, dolls, animals and hearts, to name a just a few of the designs with which nurses became familiar. The pin-cushions were not without their uses. The wise probationer would ensure that the needle was always threaded with black thread ready to undertake a hastily cobbled repair on the ladder or hole discovered in a stocking just as Matron or one of her deputies was about to do a ward round. (A sewing box was kept on every ward but this was not always readily available in moments of crisis.) The stainless steel safety pins had numerous uses, amongst them securing bandages, slings, gowns and aprons (in an emergency) and night shades. Gold pins were kept exclusively for securing mortuary sheets, always ensuring the point of the pin was pointing away from the head of the deceased.

It was probably intended that each Christmas the new pin-cushion would be donned and the old one discarded. In practice many nurses concealed a collection of pin-cushions beneath their aprons, the number to some extent being equated with status; if nothing else, a large collection of pin-cushions witnessed to the length of time their owner had been at the Royal. Sadly, in the 1950s the pin-cushions were identified as a potential source of infection and the wearing of them was prohibited.

Nurses were not the only recipients of pin-cushions. Custom decreed that sister made miniature editions for medical staff, some of whom were gallant enough to wear them on jacket lapels as they did their traditional Christmas 'round'. Miniatures were also sent to Matron. At least one matron, Miss Theodora Turner, who was in post from 1948 to 1953, is known to have displayed an entire array of pin-cushions on a screen at the entrance to her flat.

Great thought was also given, well in advance, to the themes for the ward and departmental Christmas decorations. Inevitably, Nativity scenes featured prominently and much ingenuity was needed to get appropriate illumination, bearing in mind that, in the interests of safety, no naked flames could be used. But fairy-tale and nursery-rhyme themes were also firm favourites and included Snow White and the Seven Dwarfs, Cinderella, Jack and the Beanstalk, Humpty Dumpty, The Snow Queen and The Teddy Bears' Picnic. There was plenty of scope for artistic talent. Volunteers and conscripts were enlisted from nursing, medical, paramedical and domestic staff. Lucky was the ward that could gain the support of the students from the local Art College! Convalescent patients could also be relied upon to make a useful contribution, their efforts seen as providing a form of diversional, if not occupational, therapy. The convalescent rooms were hives of industry and even patients confined to bed were to be seen gumming, stitching and folding a variety of materials into interesting shapes.

Special mention must be given to light shades. Overhead bed lights, central ward and corridor lights - normally covered with drab and strictly utilitarian bakelite shades - were transformed into things of eye-catching beauty with ingeniously invented and crafted shades, the design of which, where possible, reflected the overall ward theme.

The source of funding for the Christmas decorations and presents is worthy of note. Each ward and department received a modest allowance from the amenity funds, and receipts for every penny spent had to be presented to the Assistant Matron after Christmas. Welcome though it was, the allowance was not enough to meet even basic expenses. The author, when a ward sister, remembers spending £1 10s. (£1.50) on a tree - an essential piece of Christmas equipment - and that made quite a hole in a total allowance of £6 10s. (£6.50). Occasionally a patient donated a tree, to the great relief and gratitude of the sister. Other contributions included gifts in money and in kind from grateful patients and their relatives and were always much appreciated. Normally, nursing staff were not allowed to accept gifts, but donations for the ward at Christmas seemed to escape the notice of the administration!

In some parts of the hospital, especially in the male wards, the patients themselves thought up ways of raising Christmas funds. For example, the last patient into bed at night, or those caught smoking out of hours, might be penalised by their fellows and the 'fines' put towards the cost of the celebrations. But however imaginative the schemes, lack of funds meant that it was vital to take care of decorations so that they could be used for several years. Once the festivities were over, as many as possible were carefully wrapped and labelled ready for storage in a locked room in the attic. Access to the store could only be gained at specific times during the period immediately before Christmas. In spite of the care taken to label ward decorations clearly so that they could be reclaimed by their rightful owners the following year, it was sometimes the case that the first come were the best served!

Christmas tree lights in hospital suffered the same ills as those in private homes: there was inevitably one loose bulb or faulty connection, and much effort was needed, with the kind co-operation of the hospital electrician, to ensure a functioning set for each ward.

Having thought up a theme for decorating the ward, sister and her nurses made a list of the necessary equipment. In spite of careful recycling there were never enough decorations, and the hunt was on for extra materials. It was in this sort of preparation that the forward planners amongst the sisters came into their own. Some started very early and at the beginning of January were to be seen touring the department stores asking for discarded decorations: as a result quantities of tinsel, paper decorations, artificial Christmas trees, lanterns and other material no longer wanted by the shops found their way to the L.R.I. Many a Father Christmas and reindeer was borne along Lime Street, up London Road and Pembroke Place (if lucky, conveyed on a number 6 or 40 tram) to be secreted in the store room ready to make a surprise appearance the following year. Enterprising ward sisters also wrote to local firms to request colourful posters or cut-outs, which might be used to decorate wards. One, who wrote to Penguin Biscuits to ask for pictures of penguins was rewarded with a box of biscuits as well! And when her ward theme was 'Teddy Bears' Picnic', she asked for pictures of bears. Bear Brand Stockings sent her boxes which featured the firm's bear logo, but sadly there were no stockings in the boxes! When the author chose the Willow Pattern scene for her ward theme a Chinese patient supplied lanterns from the restaurant where he worked.

Officially, decorations could not be put up before Christmas Eve, but furtive attempts were made to get the less obvious trimmings in place earlier. Porters clothed the main corridor lights in their chosen mantels and hung the festoons of tinsel and paper decorations. They also delivered the trees to the wards and departments. There were occasions when the tree, carefully and lovingly selected, did not get to its intended destination and the irate ward sister had to make do with an inferior specimen left stranded in the courtyard with no label attached.

As in any home, decorating the tree was a 'family' affair, much enjoyed by staff and patients alike. Patients' presents were provided by the hospital and also purchased from ward funds. Some local firms provided biscuits, sweets and toiletries which made useful stocking fillers. It was difficult to assess the number of gifts required because of the fluctuations in patient numbers.

The aim was to reduce the number to a minimum over the holiday period. Planned admissions ceased during Christmas week and the medical staff tried to discharge as many patients as possible to spend Christmas in their own homes. Social circumstances were, however, taken into account and a few whose home situation was unhappy or who had no home to go to enjoyed not only the festivities, but the luxury of warmth and shelter. 'Regular customers' could also be found in the wards at Christmas. Some suffered from illnesses which necessitated frequent admission to hospital. One such was Bill (not his real name, like others in this chapter his identity has been disguised) a haemophiliac. Christmas in the community was for him a hazard, as the slightest injury could cause severe bleeding and painful haemarthroses (bleeding into the joints). The frustration of not being able to join the rough and tumble with his brothers and their friends when they had had a few drinks was more than Bill could bear and for him the ward was a haven. He was a mine of information on past hospital Christmases and delighted in telling staff and patients alike about them, a task which helped to compensate for the limitations his medical condition imposed upon him.

Another Christmas regular was Rob, whose renal rickets had arrested his growth and left him with deformed legs; he was unable to get around without a wheelchair or crutches. Like Bill, he found his physical condition a particular burden at Christmas and was sometimes more at home in the hospital environment. Barry, however, tended to be admitted to hospital during, rather than before, the festive period. He had severe diabetes mellitus which could normally be controlled with the aid of diet and insulin. He could impress doctors and nurses alike with his apparent in-depth knowledge of his condition and it was difficult to understand the reason for his crisis admissions. Barry lived with his elderly parents who, in spite of repeated counselling sessions, waited until he was slipping into a comatose state before summoning medical aid. On Christmas or Boxing Day Barry might well be seen in the ward with an intravenous 'lifeline' in place and a nurse in constant attendance. Miraculously, he always seemed to make a quick recovery and would soon be found offering fellow diabetics the questionable benefit of his advice. It was only by chance that it was discovered that Barry's relapses were usually preceded by nights out in the local hostelries, following which diet and insulin were forgotten.

Ulcerative colitis had been Ann's constant companion for many years. Prolonged medical treatment, extensive surgery and a broken marriage resulted in loss of self-esteem and hope. Christmas in hospital provided Ann with the care and attention she craved. She delighted in providing small gifts for the nursing staff and eagerly awaited the visit of her young, only son on Christmas Day.

Casualty department had its regular visitors too, including Joe and Dolly, methylated spirit drinkers, who, after stomach washouts, were assured of a bed for the night and a breakfast of tea and toast.

Perhaps the saddest cases were those whom, for one reason or another, society had rejected. The ever-present loneliness of such people became even more acute at a time when families were gathering to celebrate the joys of Christmas and their cries for help were manifested in drug overdosage. Attempts to integrate them in the 'ward family' were often unsuccessful because of their feelings of guilt and unworthiness at a time when attempted suicide carried with it a great social stigma.

There were usually more patients in medical than in surgical wards over Christmas, but when attempting to assess potential numbers allowance had to be made for emergency admissions and careful consideration was given to the 'take-in' rota, which was a system by which the different consultants and their staff took it in turns to be responsible for dealing with those who had been admitted to Casualty.

Catering, for both patients and staff, was largely carried out in the main kitchen situated in the attic on the third floor. It was a time-honoured custom, however, to prepare the jellies and trifles in the ward kitchen. And fairy cakes, mince pies and biscuits could be, and were, baked by the more culinary gifted of the nurses, in the ample stoves to be found in every ward kitchen.

No Christmas preparations would have been complete without the carol singing practices. These began a few weeks before Christmas in the hospital chapel under the direction of a senior member of the nursing staff, accompanied, initially, on the organ by a sister or probationer. (It was believed by some that ability to play the organ earned the aspiring probationer bonus points at the selection interview!)

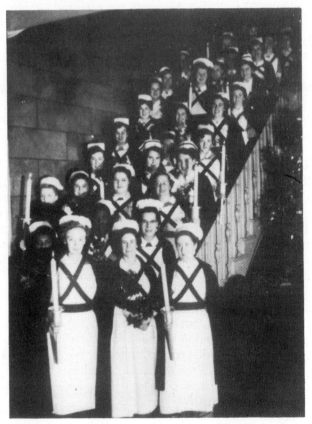

Rehearsing carols for Christmas Eve,
Liverpool Royal Infirmary, 1953.

Practices were held at the end of the day shift and senior members of the nursing staff were posted at strategic points on the route from the wards to the nurses' home, to ensure that all weary feet (clad, of course, in sensible black lace-up shoes with rubber protected medium heels) trod the corridor leading to the chapel. Every effort was made to get the choristers word and note perfect. In the present writer's time as a probationer, Sister Egerton was in charge of carol practice. She must have been one of the most enthusiastic and exacting of choir leaders. Commitment of heart and soul, as well as voice, was demanded and she frequently interrupted the carollers to remind them that 'The Herald Angels 'sing', they don't 'sin '.

At the 'dress rehearsal' cloaks were donned, lanterns lit (one between each pair of nurses) and the choir practised walking in procession, singing unaccompanied and referring only briefly to their carol sheets. The original lanterns of black cardboard and coloured cellophane paper had been made by the soldiers who had been nursed in the hospital during the First World War. They were illuminated by a battery-operated bulb and it was no mean task for the nurse carrying the lantern to keep her thumb on the button to maintain contact.

Singing in unison was not easily accomplished. As the long crocodile processed, negotiating corners and stairs - especially the spiral staircases (known as the monkey stairs) - it was possible for the leaders to be on the first verse of 'As with gladness, men of old' whilst the tail-enders rendered the last verse of 'While shepherds watched their flocks'.

By the afternoon of Christmas Eve, the ward themes were usually recognisable, having previously been kept a closely guarded secret. The patients' presents were wrapped and labelled, ready for the night nurses to distribute in makeshift stockings, pillow-slips, or decorative carrier bags, before first light. Trifles and jellies, just awaiting their finishing touches, were stored in a cool place (refrigerators were not installed in ward kitchens until the 1940s).

By 8.00 p.m., with most of the preparations completed and with all the patients cosily tucked up in bed, the day and night staff gathered round sister's desk in the middle of the ward, in

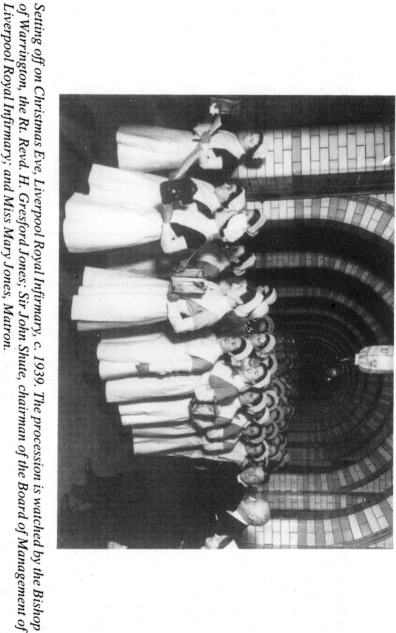

Setting off on Christmas Eve, Liverpool Royal Infirmary, c. 1939. The procession is watched by the Bishop of Warrington, the Rt. Revd. H. Gresford Jones; Sir John Shute, chairman of the Board of Management of Liverpool Royal Infirmary; and Miss Mary Jones, Matron.

readiness for the traditional evening prayers. Until well into the 1950s the main ward lights were always switched off at 8.00 p.m. and the shaded night lights and flickering flames from the well-stoked coal fires provided the only illumination. The night nurses were left to do their round of the patients, giving them their night beverages of Bournvita, Milo or (frequently lumpy) Horlicks.

The choristers amongst the day staff set off for the chapel to assemble in the carol-singing procession, the senior sisters leading and the most junior probationers bringing up the rear. Upon receiving the signal from the choir leader, the procession set off in orderly formation. It was customary for the choir to walk round each ward, pausing to complete one carol. The patients loved it and those who were able joined in the singing. It was always appreciated when a Welsh tenor lent his voice in perfect harmony. Some patients were overcome with emotion as they remembered home, family and friends. If there were very ill patients in the ward the choir remained in the corridor.

Having completed the round of the wards, the choir proceeded, weather permitting, to the courtyard between the Tropical Ward and the 'round' wards, six and twelve. Here, the choristers gathered round to sing the final carol, Silent Night. This was the most memorable and moving part of the carol evening and it was surprising just how far the voices carried as they echoed in the emptiness of the cobbled courtyard.

The, by now, hungry and thirsty members of the choir, made their way to the dining-room in the Nurses' Home, to enjoy whatever refreshments had been kept for them, before retiring weary but happy.

Meanwhile, in the wards, the night nurses continued to minister to the needs of the patients, fitting in, also, the duties of a more domestic nature. The sterilisers (most of which were situated in the wards) had to be emptied and cleaned, cups and saucers had to be washed and any soiled linen sluiced, to mention just a few of the chores. Clean bed linen was a 'must' on Christmas morning and was put out in readiness for 7.30 a.m. when the day and night staff joined forces in making the beds. Care was taken to ensure that no well-meaning patient got up to stoke the coal fires which, during the winter months, were kept burning from round about lunch-time until after the patients had all gone to bed. There was usually a good fire when the night staff reported for duty, but it was then unwise to add any more fuel as each morning the ward maid had to rake out the ashes and reset the fire. Woe betide the night nurses if the ashes were still hot when the maid arrived on duty!

Christmas morning began with the celebration of Holy Communion in the hospital chapel at 6.00 a.m. for those Anglican members of staff who wished to attend. One of the sisters then accompanied the Anglican chaplain to the wards to administer the Sacrament to the patients. The night nurses were responsible for preparing the patients who had requested Holy Communion, arranging, whenever possible, for any ambulant patients to sit round the screened bed of a non-ambulant one. Night sister 'phoned each ward in advance of the chaplain's arrival and every effort was made to ensure privacy and quietness during the short bedside service.

The Roman Catholic nurses made their way to Mass at one of the local churches. The priests made their own arrangements for giving the Sacrament to the Roman Catholic patients, the night nurses ensuring that the locker tops had been cleared and that the special Holy Communion set was available. Patients of other Christian denominations were visited by their clergy.

At 7.30 a.m., barring emergencies, all was ready for bed-making and essential cleaning to be done before sister arrived on duty at 8.00 a.m. Sister, after exchanging festive greetings with patients and staff, received the report from the night nurse and then set to work serving the breakfasts.

Cooked breakfast, usually bacon and egg, was provided on Christmas morning, although some patients, especially those from the farming areas of Wales, preferred to have their own eggs. The 'pro on kitchens' went round with a basket collecting the eggs, carefully pencilling the patient's name or bed number on the shell to ensure that each boiled egg reached its correct owner! Requests were made for alternative cooking methods and unfortunate was the 'pro' who ended up with orders for two boiled, one fried, three poached and two scrambled! Kindly ward maids, and, in later years, orderlies would sometimes lend a hand and every 'pro' appreciated the need to keep in their good books.

Sister, with white sleeves rolled down, [2] presided over the serving of breakfasts, with the 'pros' carrying the meal to each patient, stopping to feed or assist as necessary. The mood was generally festive but was more subdued when there was a terminally ill patient in the ward.

Breakfasts served, and domestic chores more or less completed, the nursing staff, in rota, went to get coffee and change their aprons. Coffee was available in the basement of the Nurses' Home on this occasion, the dining-room being declared 'out of bounds' whilst preparations were made for the nurses' Christmas dinner. Many staff, however, preferred to follow the Sunday practice (strictly against the rules!) of preparing coffee in the ward kitchen. This was a delicious brew made in a somewhat unorthodox manner. Milk, usually well-diluted, was placed in a large saucepan and ground coffee was sprinkled on the top. The infusion was brought gently to the boil and then strained through gauze into a jug. It was not unusual for the appointed coffee-maker to be called to attend to more urgent duties, and the coffee to boil over, forming an unsightly, congealed mass on the top of the stove. The perpetrator of this crime invoked the wrath and indignation, not just of sister, but more importantly, also of the ward maid. The unfortunate nurse often made reparation by cleaning the stove herself.

There was a service in the chapel on Christmas morning and those patients who were fit enough to attend were accompanied by as many nurses as could be spared. Some patients walked and some were taken in wheel-chairs which had to be manhandled down and then up the chapel steps. Apart from their night clothes and dressing-gowns, the patients were warmly wrapped in the colourful rugs of knitted squares, made by the ladies of the Linen League.

After the service the morning beverages were served and then all nursing staff attended to the patients' needs and made them comfortable, ready for dinner.

For some patients it was an opportunity to put on gifts (not infrequently new nightdresses, bed-jackets, pyjamas, dressing-gowns and slippers). The ladies made liberal use of their various toiletries. All patients wanted to look their best when the consultant staff - often accompanied by their families - the Chairman of the House Committee and, of prime importance, their own relatives and friends visited.

Serving the Christmas dinner was a truly 'family' affair, the consultant assuming the paternal role and carving the turkey. It was usual to provide an improvised apron, made from a towel to which red ribbon had hastily been stitched, to form a halter and apron strings! For those who dared, attempts were made to fashion a tall chef's hat. The bird was carved with due ceremony and served with all the trimmings; it was followed, after a suitable interval, by the plum pudding and brandy sauce.

That so special a Christmas meal was provided was largely thanks to the work of the staff in the hospital kitchen, led for many years by a housekeeping sister and later by a catering officer. Over a period of weeks, plum puddings and Christmas cakes were mixed and cooked, followed by the mince pies. Then the turkeys were dressed (in the days before the ready availability of the frozen variety!), stuffed with home-made forcemeat and surrounded by sausages. Pounds of carrots, sprouts and potatoes (for roasting and boiling) were prepared by the kitchen maids. Special diets were provided for the patients unable to eat the Christmas fare.

At a convenient time, the staff assembled near the tree to receive their pin-cushions and other small gifts. The pin-cushions were duly admired and pinned, just for the day, on the apron bibs. After

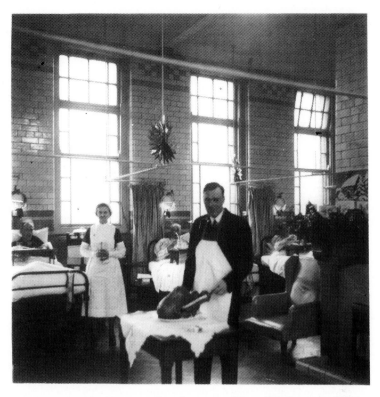

Carving the Christmas turkey, Liverpool Royal Infirmary, 1950s

Christmas they would have to be concealed under the apron. Much thought and effort had gone into the selection of a suitable gift for sister from the staff. It was usually the charge-nurse who assumed responsibility for discreetly finding out what sister would like and then buying it.

When the meal and the ceremonies which followed it were over, the ward was closed whilst nursing procedures were carried out and then the patients were left in peace for a nap before visiting time. The staff had their meal in relays, usually in a room adjacent to the ward.

The ward kitchen continued to be the scene of much activity, for, as soon as the dishes had been washed, work commenced on setting the trolley ready for afternoon tea. Each patient could invite two visitors to share whatever delicacies were available. Sandwiches usually replaced the normal bread and jam tea and there were jellies, trifles, mince pies and Christmas cake. Inevitably, a few patients had no visitors. Although some limited public transport was available on Christmas Day, for some the journey was too long or too complicated to enable them to visit. Other patients had no family or friends with whom they could share the joys of the festive season, and initially they sought refuge under cover of the bedclothes or buried their heads in books or magazines. But they need not have tried to escape from loneliness, for the warm-hearted Liverpudlians ensured that there were visitors at every bed, unless a patient genuinely wanted to be alone. It was generally a noisy, happy occasion.

During the course of the afternoon, the nursing staff took it in turn to visit other wards and departments to cast a critical eye over the decorations and pin-cushions of their colleagues.

Before the last of the patients' visitors had left, the staff had begun the late afternoon and early evening treatments, for soon all, with the exception of sister, would be going off duty to change into clean uniform in readiness for the nurses' Christmas Dinner, which was also attended by the night staff. The dinner was a formal affair served by the senior nursing staff with the maids in their best uniform waiting at table. The highlight of the meal was when one of the longest serving maids bore aloft the flaming plum pudding, decorated with a sprig of holly. Ladylike cheers were permitted on this occasion! The replete nurses then made their way to the Rankin Room and the gaily decorated tree, on and beneath which were gifts for each nurse, Matron, assisted by her deputies, playing the role of Father Christmas.

In the wards the sisters continued, unaided, to care for the patients. Ambulant patients, especially in the male wards, were very supportive, attending to the minor, but very essential needs of their fellow sufferers. (It was a source of great amazement to some patients that sister could, and would, make drinks and give out bed-pans and urinals!) The report was written, the night drinks dispensed, the night nurses' table or cabinet set and the final round of the patients made. This was one of the most poignant moments, for, almost without exception, patients were appreciative of all the efforts made to keep the traditions of Christmas. Some felt it had been the next best thing to being at home with loved ones, whilst others had experienced rare moments of true fellowship.

The night staff arrived on duty and sister slipped away to join her peers in the Sisters' Residence or to meet up, if only briefly, with family or friends.

Boxing Day was relatively quiet and staff got some off-duty, which in later years amounted to a half day. By now the decorations had begun to lose their glitter and the Christmas Tree its pine needles, and all the staff braced themselves for the influx of planned and emergency admissions.

The sisters could still anticipate their Christmas dinner held on Boxing Night. Like the nurses, the sisters attended their dinner in uniform. Some in the mid-1950s thought that this practice was outmoded and the issue was put to the vote at a sisters' meeting. An overwhelming majority voted in favour of mufti being worn, but democracy crumbled when the powerful minority insisted that tradition be upheld!

On the Great Night, the sisters assembled in Matron's flat to sip sherry served by her maid, before descending the stairs to the dining-room. A special, luxurious feature of the dinner was the champagne provided by Mr Norman Roberts, who was a senior orthopaedic surgeon. It was unwise to make an enemy of Matron's maid, who recharged the glasses of those who found favour. The sisters also went to the sitting room to receive their gifts from the tree.

During the lifetime of the great benefactor, Mr Walter Harding, another noteworthy event was eagerly anticipated. After Christmas, all the nurses were taken to the pantomime, half on each of two consecutive nights. They were escorted on one night by

71

Matron and on the other by her assistant. Dressed in full uniform, the nurses walked in an orderly crocodile down Pembroke Place and London Road to the Empire Theatre, where Mr Harding had reserved seats for them on the front rows of the stalls. To add to the enjoyment, Mr Harding also provided boxes of chocolates. The sisters continued to have a night out at the pantomime, well into the post-World War II years.

The celebrations would not have been complete without the nurses' Christmas Dance. This event appears to have been organised by various individual groups of nurses and held in different venues, but best remembered must surely be the dances attended in the out-patients' department. This was a formal, if not formidable, setting for a most formal occasion. Senior nursing staff were expected to attend this event in uniform and they sat, in a row, in solitary splendour. Names and addresses of nurses' partners had been submitted to Matron's office in advance of the dance, and on the appointed day at the appointed hour, the nurses, in modest evening dress, lined up to present their partners to Matron. Dancing on the terrazzo floor was fraught with hazard, especially when it came to negotiating the basement sky-lights! And once in the 'dance hall' couples were expected to remain for the evening. Matron or one of her deputies sat near the door, not actually barring the exit, but making it clear that note would be taken of those who left early. But in spite of all the restrictions, a good time was had by all.

Needless to say, various staff groups organised their own celebrations, many of which would have been frowned upon by those in authority had they known of them. Several nurses crept 'over the bridge' to parties in the doctors' residence. A few unfortunates were caught by night sister, but, after being turned back, generally escaped with a caution.

Much has changed over the years as more and more nurses have become non-resident and attitudes have changed. Also, in the interests of saving money, as many wards as possible are now closed over the Christmas holiday period. But it is to be hoped that many of the traditions will never die.

Notes

[1] B.Eaglesfield and B.M. Phillips, *Liverpool Royal Infirmary Nurses' Training School 1862-1962* (Liverpool, 1962)
[2] Sisters and charge nurses wore long, detachable, white sleeves, secured to the short sleeves of the dress by safety pins. It was imperative that the sleeves were worn correctly at all times. They were rolled up for many nursing and domestic procedures, but swiftly rolled down and their cuffs buttoned for the matron's and doctor's rounds, serving meals, taking patients' temperatures and administering medicines. They were removed altogether when carrying out 'last offices' (laying out the dead).

Chapter 6
Behind Closed Doors
Helen Brett

Well-documented references to the early days of theatre nursing are almost non-existent. Indeed, it can be argued that this particular branch of nursing is a child of the mid-twentieth century. That some nurses were employed in theatres in the past is not in question, but mention of individuals such as Sister MacBride, who worked at the Liverpool Royal Infirmary from 1880 until 1908 and as a theatre sister worked with many well-known surgeons such as Frank Thomas Paul, is rare. It certainly should not be presumed that she was a theatre sister/nurse in today's sense of the words but rather that she supervised the running of the operating theatre whenever it was required and whatever the category of staff employed there. Quite often such a nurse would be the sister in charge of the surgical ward and would double as a theatre sister when needed. This practice was very common in those hospitals where the operating theatre was adjacent to the ward and continued well into the twentieth century in many instances, particularly in specialised branches of surgery such as ophthalmics and gynaecology.

In the nineteenth century there were few purpose-built operating theatre suites such as those in modern hospitals, and collection of such suites into departments was virtually unknown. It was only when the work of Louis Pasteur, Ignaz P. Semmelweiss, Lord Lister and others began to have its effect and antiseptics were introduced into the surgical world that the need for a special environment in which surgeons could work was recognised. These times were quickly followed by the development of aseptic practice and by those techniques which aimed to give the surgeon and his team as clean an operating field as possible. It was then that special rooms began to be set aside for the purpose.

The present-day theatre nurse, who is trained to give care to the patients pre- and post-operatively, to prepare supplies and instruments and to assist the surgeons and the anaesthetist is a far cry from the nurse in charge of the instruments and the theatre of the early days of surgery. It was far more common in those days to have male assistants fulfilling this role, cleaning the room and furniture, sharpening and oiling the instruments and holding down the struggling patient. Surgery was more often the treatment of desperation - a failure by the physicians to cure or made necessary as the result of an accident or violence such as war. It was regarded as the poor relation and did not 'merit' the services of trained nurses.

What has happened between the days of people like Sister MacBride and the theatre nurse of today merits the attention of a skilled researcher before memories have faded and evidence of that past has disappeared. This century has seen technical advances beyond most people's wildest dreams and with such advances has been the development of operating theatre design and practice necessitating staff with skills that are equally sophisticated and special. However, the following pages may give a little insight into life in an operating theatre in the early days of the National Health Service.

Between the two world wars, both of which had far-reaching effects upon surgical techniques and the status of the surgeon, came the beginning of theatre nursing as a separate discipline, requiring additional skills to those of a bedside nurse.

The effects of the Second World War were even more dramatic, with the introduction of the sulpha drugs, antibiotics, the development of both blood transfusion techniques and the science of anaesthesia. All these, and more besides, have led to the incredible surgical feats which are practised daily in our hospitals in the 1990s. Side by side with such advances has been the further development of theatre nursing as a specialised branch of nursing, whose skills demand not only assistance to the surgeon but also the ability to care for the patient within the operating department and the ability to manage the provision of supplies and to provide the training to ensure the staff of the future.

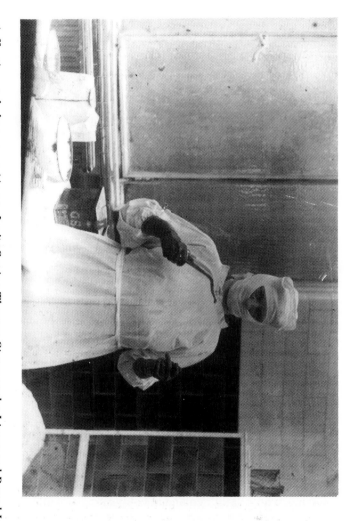

Sister Ivy Benn (affectionately known as 'Aunty Ivy'), Senior Theatre Sister at the Liverpool Royal Infirmary, who retired in 1952.

To some extent, the 1939-45 War had the effect of making time stand still in the civilian hospitals. Money, staff and equipment were needed elsewhere and some of the techniques used also stood still, so that people who began nursing in the late 1940s, as the author did, had the dubious distinction, on some occasions, of working in what amounted to a 'time warp.' The following are some personal reminiscences before the advent of the modern operating theatres, theatre nursing courses, C.S.S.D.s, T.S.S.U.s [1] and the age of disposable equipment and the Health and Safety at Work Act.

Staffing for the four theatres of the Liverpool Royal Infirmary consisted of two theatre sisters, four senior nurses, four student nurses, one night nurse (a 3rd year student nurse) and two theatre porters.

Two of the four theatres which took the lion's share of the surgery had been opened in 1902 by Sir Frederick Treves - a very famous name in surgical history; the other two - known as the 'new theatres', officially opened by their Royal Highnesses the Duke and Duchess of York in 1925, and originally designed to cater for gynaecology and obstetrics, were, by the late 1940s, rapidly proving inadequate to cope with the enormous changes in surgical technique which were then beginning.

When recording the impressions of the late 1940s, it is of the old theatres that one thinks and so it is perhaps more appropriate to describe those as a setting into which can be put the next few pages rather than to describe the so-called 'new theatres' or Larrinaga theatres (named after a benefactor of the Liverpool Royal Infirmary) which eventually bridged the gap between the old way of life and the new.

Each of the old twin theatres operated independently of the other and in design was a perfect mirror image of its twin. However, as the senior surgeon operated in Theatre 1, the junior surgeon and his team working in Theatre 2 often had to make do with the older instruments and equipment and the least experienced staff of all categories. Within each theatre was housed everything that was needed for the whole operating list. On one side of the room were the shallow stone sinks where the surgeon and his medical and nursing team scrubbed their hands and arms before putting on the sterile gowns and gloves which were set out close by. On the opposite wall - but still in the operating theatre - was a deep sink where the instruments were scrubbed clean by hand after use and re-assembled in trays to await sterilisation by boiling. Here too was a flushing hopper sink where soiled linen was sluiced clean with water and where the disposal of fluids of one sort and another took place. Alongside were the boilers used for sterilising the instruments, stainless steel bowls and trays, jugs and other metal or glass equipment that might be needed (a method which is now acknowledged as inadequate to destroy all the pathogenic organisms contaminating the used instruments and equipment). Ranged along the tiled walls were the copper or stainless steel drums (boxes) in which the sterile towels, gowns, dressings, gloves and so on were stored. And at the far end of the theatre were two large water tanks which provided cold and hot sterile water. These were a welcome addition installed in the 1950s, but unfortunately, while they ensured a safer water supply, they also added to the steam from the boilers which belched forth into the theatre during the operating list. Quite often it was not just steam which poured forth as the poor little probationer nurse - usually known as the 'runner' and often the only person in the theatre not in sterile garb - would turn the heat up on the boilers and then be called to open the sterile drums, tie the gowns of the surgical team, help to lift the unconscious patient on to the table, mop the floor, pick up the soiled swabs, answer the telephone and even put the kettle on for sister's tea, only to remember too late about the boilers and find that boiling water was pouring out over the floor to add to the general air of dampness already present. Turning off the taps whilst boiling water cascaded over the sides of the boiler was just another hazard of being the 'pro' or runner in theatre!

Reference to the steam-laden atmosphere is particularly important as there was no form of ventilation in the theatres, other than by covering the open window with a sheet of gauze to keep out the birds and bees and, in the middle of summer, by leaving the

78

doors open and placing a folding screen in front of the gap! On visiting days, it gave the patients' visitors an insight into the hidden world of the operating theatre and often a row of eyes could be seen peering over and through the screens. This practice of leaving doors and windows open was by no means unique and, whilst not always so public, was commonplace throughout the country at that time. Theatre ventilation was very much in its infancy and few hospitals boasted a properly ventilated operating theatre.

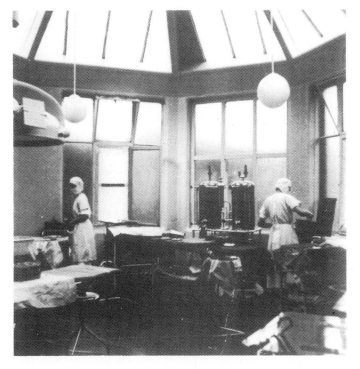

Theatre 1, Liverpool Royal Infirmary in the 1950s, showing nurses dressing the theatre in readiness for the afternoon operating list.

And lastly, at the back of the theatre was the glass-fronted cupboard which housed the instruments when not in use.

A further factor which affected the comfort, health and safety of the staff, was the roof of the theatre which was almost totally made of glass. At the time of its planning and building in 1902 this glazed roof would have maximised the use of day-light to assist the surgeon in his task, but in the early days of the Health Service, when lighting was already quite sophisticated, it only helped to make the conditions in the summer like working in a greenhouse and in the winter, when the steam-laden air met the cold glass, like working in a house with a leaky roof. Was it any wonder that it was difficult to recruit nurses to work in theatres? The Medical and Nursing Committee Minutes of 1900 show that this problem existed even then.

Each theatre had a small ante-room where the patients were usually anaesthetized lying on a trolley and from where they would be wheeled in to the theatre and lifted on to the operating table. It was a task which required the help of all the theatre staff; and the reverse process, when the patient was returned to the trolley to be taken back to the ward, also necessitated the strength of several people. Whatever their status or age, everybody was expected to lift the unconscious patient and the one vivid memory of these occasions was of the senior surgeon, himself one of the four lifters, counting 'One, two, three, LIFT -' and urging everyone to 'keep the back straight'.

Each day began with the preparation of the theatre - all surfaces were carbolised - the very word is a hang-over from Lister's day, and entailed washing down all the walls and furniture with phenol solution. Cheatle forceps were boiled up and then immersed in an antiseptic solution for the rest of the day. These were used to lift sterile instruments and utensils out of the large boilers and to dress the instrument tables with sterile waterproofs and sterile 'carbolic towels'. Lister again.

Before the installation of tanks for sterile water, hot sterile water was obtained by dipping jugs into the boilers - and many burned fingers resulted from the practice! Cold water came from a water filter made of porous stone which was attached to the mains water supply.

Instruments - one set per theatre - were boiled and subsequently put on the sterile instrument trolley at the beginning of the list - and there they stayed. Those required for the particular operation were lifted off using cheatle forceps and placed on the Mayo stand 2 by the scrub nurse or theatre sister. Once the case had begun, the table itself was never touched by the nurse's hands, gloved though they were. Everything was handled with forceps in order to keep the main supply of instruments 'sterile'. No thought was given to contamination by the air itself!

Lengths of catgut were provided in sealed, glass tubes and very scarce they were too. Needles were stored in lysol and threaded with the catgut by the scrub nurse, as required. Some of the catgut was not commercially sterilised but was wound into coils by the theatre staff, put into jars and left to soak in a solution of iodine or alcohol prior to use.

Towels and waterproof sheeting were folded and packed into copper drums prior to being sterilised by steam under pressure. This was all done by the nurses.

Rubber gloves were powdered and packed before sterilisation, again by the nurses, and at the end of the operating list were washed, boiled and hung out to dry. They were then tested for holes by the night nurse. Any gloves with holes were patched - usually a weekend task - for use later by the surgeons' assistants and students. All the gloves were powdered, paired and re-packed for sterilisation - whether new or re-used. At the end of the daily packing session, the nurses would emerge covered in white chalk - eyebrows, eyelashes and no doubt lungs!

Swabs and abdominal packs were made with first quality gauze by the senior theatre sister and her assistant. All were hand-sewn. Abdominal packs were washed, sterilised and used again. Swabs were not. Their constant supply was one of the 'head-aches' of being a senior theatre nurse. Gauze was hard to come by and so were the patients who did the sewing! Each morning a senior theatre nurse would sally forth to the female wards - bearing bundles of hand-folded gauze swabs, sewing needles and thread, on the look-out for likely seamstresses amongst the patients. Wiser, long-stay patients often would feign sleep as soon as the theatre nurse appeared, leaving the hapless new patients to bear the brunt!

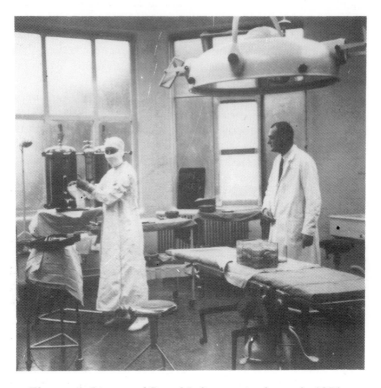

Theatre 1, Liverpool Royal Infirmary in the early 1950s, ready for the afternoon list to begin.

And then there were the radiation hazards! In those years, little attention was paid to the dangers of working with radio-active materials and X-rays. No protective clothing was worn and the theatre sister would sit down with a collection of radium needles which had been delivered in a lead-lined box from the Radium Institute and thread the radium with anchoring threads using her bare hands. This often took half an hour or more. X-rays taken during surgery often involved the surgeon or scrub nurse holding the unexposed film whilst the machine was operated.

One of the most important tasks of the student nurse was to put out the white suits which the surgeons wore. It was more than her life was worth to put ready trousers which did not fit or suits with buttons missing. Each surgeon had his own white twill suits made to measure. In addition, sterilised long-sleeved cotton gowns were worn by the surgical teams in the operating theatre, but there was one senior surgeon at the Liverpool Royal Infirmary who insisted on wearing the sterile white, cotton aprons and sleeves which in his young days his chief had worn. This same surgeon would not allow the use of the antibiotics, relaxant drugs or intra-venous fluids then in general use.

Many of the operating lists in those days began at 1.00 p.m. - a hangover from pre-N.H.S. days when the consultants had honorary posts and gave their time after seeing their private patients in the morning. So as well as preparing instruments during the morning, theatre staff also got the theatres ready for the day's list. Bowls, utensils and instruments were boiled and tables laid out in readiness. Rarely, emergencies would be carried out. Then at 1.00 p.m. it all began. As soon as each operation was over, the unconscious patient was returned to the ward to lie alongside other such patients and await his recovery to consciousness. In a busy ward, where the nurses were generally caring for patients, serving meals, interviewing relatives and taking patients to and from theatres, X-ray departments and so on it was not possible for post-operative patients to receive the care they experience today in recovery wards. Once all the operations were finished, every instrument and bowl that had been used was cleaned with scouring powder and all the gloves and waterproofs washed and hung out to dry. Soiled linen was rinsed and counted before being sent to the laundry. Walls were washed down and floors flooded with buckets full of disinfectants - the highlight of the cleaning-up process and a marvellous way of getting rid of all the frustrations of the day along with the dirt. All this was done by the nurses, who remained on duty until the work was finished.

Cleaning instruments was a chore, but it could also be a wonderful way of learning their names and function; re-stocking catgut jars and needle pots was an equally good method of learning the types and gauges of catgut and sizes and shapes of needles. The student nurses were really pairs of hands then - very little time was given over to actual teaching and very rarely was a probationer allowed to scrub up but, in spite of that, some did find it sufficiently rewarding to want to work in theatres, once their final examinations were over.

Those early post-war years, which were also the early years of the National Health Service, were followed by what one might call the years of 'surgical liberation'. The late 1950s and the 1960s, when good anaesthesia, antibiotics and so on, together with some relaxation in the availability of supplies, meant that the green light went on so far as the surgeon was concerned. It was an enormously exciting time. But there were still shortages of staff and resources and the buildings were inadequate to deal with the work-load and the complexities of modern surgical and anaesthetic techniques, and it was not long before a new awareness of the link between post-operative mortality and morbidity and such working conditions began to have its effect.

Then came the purpose-built operating departments, C.S.S.D.s, T.S.S.U.s, anaesthetic departments and the demand for better training and standards for the rapidly expanding staff - professional and non-professional - who were needed to run such departments. Theatre nurses had to become concerned directly with patient care as the barriers went up and what evolved was infinitely superior to what had existed before.

No doubt, somewhere amongst the dusty records, held all over the city, there are references to nurses working in operating theatres in the last century and, no doubt, there are still nurses living on Merseyside today who can recall tales of operating days related to them when they were young. There will not be many because theatre nurses always were, and still are, a very scarce resource. To call them an endangered species would not be an exaggeration at any time in their history; today it could be regarded as a fact.

The links with the past are very tenuous indeed and grow more so as the months go by. Perhaps it is already too late to record this interesting and important chapter in the history of nursing.

Notes

[1] Central Sterile Supply Units and Theatre Sterile Supply Units are departments within the hospital which are similar to small factories where sterile goods, including surgical clothing, gowns and patient drapes, instrument sets etc are sterilised for ward and theatre use. The autoclaves, or steam pressure sterilisers, hot air ovens etc. are situated here and the departments are staffed by trained personnel.

[2] A cantilevered stand holding instruments which is placed over the patient near to the surgeon and the scrub nurse.

Chapter 7

Reflections on a Nurses' League

Betty Hoare

Today a Nurses' League is usually an organisation providing an opportunity for keeping in touch with friends and colleagues and with the Nurse Training School, and student nurses may be surprised to know that sixty years ago the Annual Reunion of a Nurses' League was a prestigious occasion attended by civic dignitaries, and its proceedings were reported in the local press.[1] Moreover, the League was also involved in national and international affairs.

At the Liverpool Royal Infirmary, the Annual Reunion of the Nurses' League began with a service in the hospital chapel when an address was given by a specially invited preacher. Then followed a business meeting in the hospital lecture theatre, the highlight of which was always the report by the Honorary Secretary, containing news of members. Afterwards, there was a chance to chat to friends and colleagues over a cup of tea in the Nurses' Home, and then to visit wards and departments, which welcomed members and official guests.

As a member of the Liverpool Royal Infirmary Nurses' League, I first became interested in its development in connection with tracing the history of the Nurses' Training School.[2] It became clear that the establishment of a Nurses' League had been an important first step in the development of professional nursing. The first League to be formed was that of St Bartholomew's Nurses in London in 1899. In the same year the International Council of Nurses was founded, but for British nurses to be represented internationally a national representative body was needed. In 1904 the National Council of Nurses of the United Kingdom was set up as a federation of the few nursing organisations, including nurses' leagues, which existed a the time. This development reflected a growing interest in professionalism and in due course it was to encourage the establishment of nurses' leagues throughout the country.

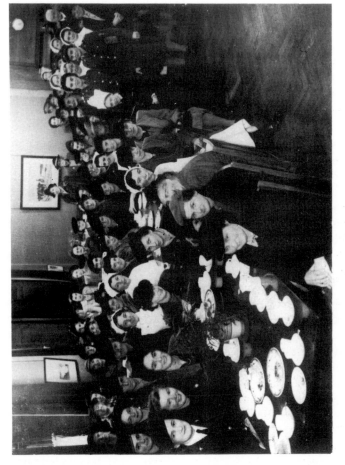

An Annual Reunion in the Nurses' Home during the Second World War.

The Liverpool Royal Infirmary Training School Nurses' League was inaugurated in 1933 by Miss Mary Jones, the Matron of the Royal Infirmary and Lady Superintendent of the Nurse Training School. Invitations to a meeting on the third Saturday in October were sent to past and present members of the nursing staff. It was clearly a successful occasion. Older nurses were asked to give talks about their experiences in training, and one of them, Miss Bates, described how she had worked for ten months before having her first day off. She also contrasted the amenities available for nurses in 1933 with those provided in her day, recalling that she and her fellow nurses had had no sitting rooms in which to relax, only what was called the Day Room, whose only decoration was a series of anatomy charts.

Miss Margaret Haynes also accepted an invitation to the inaugural meeting. She had trained as a general nurse at the Royal Infirmary, following training as a fever nurse at the Liverpool Fever Hospital in Grafton Street, and by 1933 she had returned to the Fever Hospital as a ward sister. As a probationer at the Liverpool Royal Infirmary she had been paid a salary of £16 per annum, in quarterly instalments. Nurses were allowed one day off a month and a half-day from 2.00 p.m. each week. Classes and lectures were arranged, some of them being given by Miss Jones, the Matron, who was interested in pharmacology. In addition to classes and lectures, each probationer kept a chart of practical experience, recording the nursing procedures learned and observed in the wards and departments. In 1927, Sister Darroch was appointed as the first Teaching Sister and two years later a Preliminary Training School (P.T.S.) was opened. This innovation meant that a number of probationers would begin their training together as a set. Previously a new probationer had been seen by her colleagues for the first time as a strange face at breakfast and her theoretical training would be fitted into courses already running. The Introductory Course in the P.T.S. lasted for eight weeks and the fee for the course - which included board, tuition and laundry - was £5, payable by the probationer on accepting a place in the School. Each candidate had to supply her own indoor uniform, with the exception of the dresses, which were provided by the hospital. Following the course, the probationers had to work on the wards for two months before signing an agreement to continue in the service of the hospital for four years.

Although Miss Haynes did not have the advantage of the P.T.S. herself, her training appeared to her to be well-organised and she considered that she and her contemporaries were well-prepared for their examinations and future nursing careers, her dominant memory being of a very happy time during which lifelong friendships developed.

The records of the League meetings are incorporated into the League Book, published every year. Each includes the reports of the Honorary Secretary and Treasurer and details of the Annual Reunion, together with items of interest about members. The first indication of interest in international affairs is found in the report of the Annual Reunion of 1937. Sister Darroch, Sister Tutor and Honorary Secretary of the Nurses' League, had represented the League at the Eighth International Congress of Nurses held in London earlier that year, and had attended the service at St Paul's Cathedral, where the Archbishop of Canterbury had given the address. Thirty-two countries had been represented, and of particular concern at the time was the protection of the title 'nurse'. Miss Cochrane, Matron of the Charing Cross Hospital in London, had spoken on the subject, insisting 'We must be careful that the practical side of nursing is sufficiently guarded in our curriculum. We must ensure that nursing education does not pass out of our hands. We must maintain our independence and government.' She had further stressed that only State Registered Nurses should nurse the sick: 'Nurses should not have to undergo years of training and then find their work undertaken by untrained women.'

Opportunities to debate such issues were provided by the International Council of Nurses every four years, when a Congress was held, each meeting hosted by a different country. Brief reports from these International Congresses were submitted by the League delegates and included in the League Books. Representation continued in this way until 1963, when the National

Council of Nurses amalgamated with the Royal College of Nursing, which then became the official representative body, with membership on an individual basis and not through League membership. Thus for thirty years the Liverpool Royal Infirmary Nurses' League had provided an opportunity for professional representation. Membership of the R.C.N., however, had also been encouraged so that with the transition interest in international nursing affairs continued as before.

The personal aspect of the Nurses' League is demonstrated in letters from members, published in the League Books. These invariably contain reminiscences and several occasions have provided opportunities for recalling earlier experiences - in particular the centenary of the Nurses' Training School in 1962, the Golden Jubilee of the Nurses' League in 1983 and the fifty-year commemoration of the Second World War in 1989.

Reminiscences from Dorothy C. Wisnom (née Pillars) are included in the Golden Jubilee Book of 1983. Her first day at the Royal in October 1936 coincided with the Annual Reunion of the Nurses' League, and as the nurses gathered the new probationer was filled with awe and envy. Dorothy Wisnom was one of a set of twelve nurses to enter the Preliminary Training School that October. She recalled that their rooms were on the fifth floor of the Nurses' Home and it was there that they battled for the first time with their uniform, before entering the classroom with its ennobling motto over the door: 'Enter ye to learn. Go forth to serve.'

From the P.T.S. they were each assigned to a ward the day after the King's abdication, an event which stayed in their memories long after the impact of their first day of proper nursing had faded. Dorothy Wisnom remembered the expressions of disapproval voiced by Christie, the hospital joiner, as he toured the wards with his long ladder.

As well as facing the demands of working on the wards, the new probationers of 1936 had to steel themselves for their first interview with Matron, Miss Mary Jones. She was a tiny, dynamic figure with a tremendous presence, who firmly pointed out to the new probationers that they would not be able to take holidays when they chose, nor off-duty to suit their convenience. 'The patient comes first,' she explained.

Probationer nurses did night-duty for three months at a time. Each evening they were given their 'take-aways', enamel dishes containing the raw ingredients for their night's snack, which they had to cook themselves. Before they started work, night sister led the nurses in prayer: 'Preserve and defend us from all perils and dangers of this night...' She may not have been aware that for some of those standing round her, with heads bowed, the greatest danger they anticipated was that of being discovered giving a cup of tea to the resident doctor!

During the Second World War the Infirmary maintained its service to the city, despite bombing and the need to receive casualties from the forces overseas. The League Book of 1989 contains memories of those years. Miss Rebecca Haynes was Assistant Home Sister. She recalled that the basement of the Nurses' Home was equipped as an air-raid shelter and each member of staff was provided with a straw palliasse and a blanket. Instructions were given on the use of a stirrup pump, in case of fire; this was not a difficult procedure, but it caused some amusement. In the event of an air-raid warning all resident nursing staff went down to the shelter, where a roll-call was taken. The Home Sisters had to check the rooms of all those nurses and maids who had not answered the roll-call. At the sound of the 'All clear' there was a general exodus from the shelter as everyone thankfully made their way back to their beds. Although there were some particularly noisy nights, when enemy aircraft were active over Liverpool, morale amongst staff was high. The hospital was bombed on several occasions, but the Nurses' Home suffered only slight damage from the blast.

In the League Books of the that period there are letters from members serving in the forces overseas. Miss D.F. Egerton wrote on 18 May 1943 from the Middle East: 'We have been terribly busy since we followed the advancing Eighth Army to this much fought-over town. Our hospital is about twenty minutes' walk from the town and was previously used as a barracks. It had been left by our enemies in an indescribably filthy state and sanitary arrangements deliberately disorganised. Before we had thoroughly cleaned the place or were nearly ready, huge convoys of wounded began to arrive and we somehow managed to achieve a certain degree of asepsis and to make our patients reasonably comfortable.'

Nurses serving abroad were specially mentioned later that year in the local press report of the Annual Reunion. Two hundred members came to the meeting from all parts of the country, and of the total membership, fifty-five were serving abroad, three being prisoners of war in the Far East.

However, most probationers were more concerned with the demands of training than with the activities of the Nurses' League and it was only on the day of the reunion that there was any real awareness of its activities. But the reunion was clearly a special event. In the Nurses' Home preparations were made and from mid-day onwards early arrivals greeted each other in the hospital entrance hall. Chattering groups of friends made their way to the chapel, and even there the buzz of conversation continued. Seated in the choir pews were the ward and departmental sisters in uniform, and greeting the members at the chapel entrance stood the sister tutors, also in uniform. The chapel gradually became silent as Matron and the clergy entered and the service began. In the wards, those who were on duty had been exhorted by the sisters to see that everything was kept tidy. The patients were as intrigued as the nurses when, later in the afternoon, League members came into the hospital to take an affectionate look at their old haunts. 'Do you remember?' was repeated many times as, with their friends, they wandered round the wards and chatted to patients and nurses.

In the early years of the Nurses' League, all nursing staff were resident. As Eileen Brown (née Glencross) wrote in the 1987 League Book, 'Living in meant companionship. There was always someone to unburden oneself to, to laugh or cry with. We

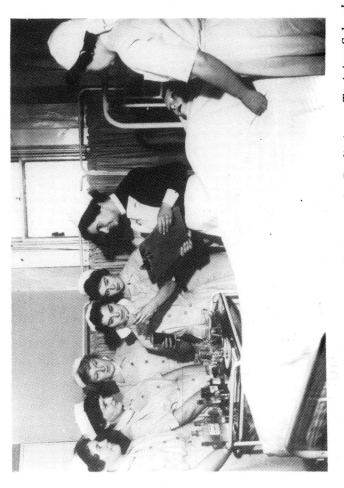

Student nurses learning how to administer medicines at the Preliminary Training School, The United Liverpool Hospitals, late 1950s. The students' caps signify the hospital to which they belonged. 'Mrs Brown', the model 'patient', had formerly been in the P.T.S. at the Liverpool Royal Infirmary.

aired our grievances to each other - the quality of the food, the disadvantages of split duties and, worst of all, having to attend lectures in our free time.' A strong community spirit was engendered that in retrospect compensated for the restrictions. Accommodation for nurses was available in the Nurses' Home although ward sisters lived in bed-sitting rooms adjacent to their wards. This arrangement ensured the total commitment of the sister to her patients, although her presence when she was officially off-duty was generally seen as a mixed blessing to the ward nurses. There were, however, signs of change.

As early as 1938 it was reported at a League meeting that there was a scheme for amalgamating the four voluntary, general hospitals in Liverpool, namely the Royal Infirmary, the Royal Southern Hospital, the David Lewis Northern Hospital and the Stanley Hospital to form The United Liverpool Hospitals. This followed a proposal for a single teaching hospital in Liverpool, which was first put forward in 1933. Subsequently, national changes in the administration of the hospital services, were brought about by the introduction of the National Health Service. The League reports mention especially the changes affecting nurse education. The requirements of the General Nursing Council for England and Wales meant an increase in the length of the P.T.S. from eight weeks to eleven weeks in 1950 and the following year a study block system was introduced. It also became necessary for arrangements to be made so that student nurses spent time away from the Royal to gain ear, nose and throat; ophthalmic, and paediatric nursing experience.

A significant step was taken by the Board of Governors of The United Liverpool Hospitals when a Preliminary Training School to serve the constituent schools of nursing was opened at Woolton Manor in March 1954. This large house had been a convalescent home, frequently mentioned in the records of the Royal Infirmary. It was adapted to provide a school for eighty student nurses, together with residential accommodation for the introductory course period. The framed inscription 'Enter ye to learn. Go forth to serve' from the classroom of the Royal Infirmary was put over the door of one of the classrooms.

This was in fact a move towards the establishment of a single school of nursing within The United Liverpool Hospitals. At the annual reunions members were kept informed as changes were made which affected the Nurses' Training School. In 1961 arrangements were made for the schemes of nurse training for the Royal Infirmary, the Royal Southern Hospital and the David Lewis Northern Hospital - the Stanley Hospital having already closed - to follow unified systems of study blocks. This was to avoid practical difficulties when the single school of nursing opened in 1968 in the Hospital College. This College building was in the first phase of the Medical Teaching Centre which was to include the proposed single teaching hospital, eventually opened in 1978 and now known as the Royal Liverpool University Hospital. With the opening of this hospital the three remaining general hospitals of The United Liverpool Hospitals closed.

The nursing profession has been greatly affected by the changes in society over the years. Following the Second World War, greater educational opportunities brought about increased alternative career options for women, and nursing, once a traditional female profession, had for some time also offered equal opportunities to men. Advances in medical science and technology have meant changes in the pattern of care and treatment for patients in hospital. All these factors and more have combined to create circumstances in which the traditional pattern of nurse training is no longer considered appropriate. Theoretical training and practical experience, once inextricably linked, have been separated.

Nurse education is now to be found within institutions of higher education. In Liverpool, the first reported link with the University was noted at the ninth Annual Reunion of the Nurses' League in October 1942, when members were told that an Honorary Degree of Master of Arts had been conferred that year on Miss Mary Jones, President of the League and Matron of the Royal Infirmary, by Lord Derby, Chancellor of the University of Liverpool. Nearly thirty years later, Miss Jones herself reported at the thirty-seventh Annual Reunion that the Board of Gover-

H.R.H. Princess Alexandra presents the prizes on the occasion of the centenary of the Liverpool Royal Infirmary Nurses' Training School, 1962.

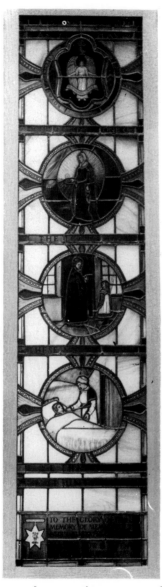

The Memorial Window, dedicated by the Bishop of Bath and Wells at the Annual Reunion in October 1954. Designed by Miss Joan Howson, it was given by members of the Nurses' League in memory of nursing colleagues. The window is now in the chapel of the Royal Liverpool University Hospital.

nors of The United Liverpool Hospitals and the Faculty of Science of the University had agreed to establish a course leading to State Registration (S.R.N.) and a Bachelor of Science degree. Thus nurse education in Liverpool took its first step towards the establishment of a University Department of Nursing.

At the fifty-fifth Reunion in 1988, it was announced that Kate Morle, a member of the Nurses' League, had been appointed the first Professor of Nursing at the University of Liverpool.

Inevitably the changes in the organisation of nurse training have meant that after 1970 newly qualified nurses were no longer eligible for membership of the Liverpool Royal Infirmary Nurses' League. Nevertheless, League members continue to meet for an Annual Reunion on the third Saturday of each October and a League Book continues to be published. From the perspective of the 1990s, the League can be seen as a link with the sources of professional standards and values, while the records provide a treasure trove of experiences, reflecting the history of nursing in a particular place at a particular time.

There were many nurses' leagues throughout the country which all played their part in the development of the profession. It is, however, the personal aspect which still endures and which is embodied in the prayer which used to be said every Sunday in the chapel of the Liverpool Royal Infirmary:

'Remember, O Lord, we beseech Thee, the work of all nurses throughout the world, especially those members, past and present, of this Hospital.

Grant that their influence, wherever they may be, may uplift mankind to a higher level, and also that their skill, sympathy and patience may alleviate pain and suffering. Guide, we pray Thee, their goings out and comings in, and foster among them always the spirit of fellowship and love. Through Jesus Christ our Lord.'

Notes

[1] *Liverpool Echo*, 18 October 1943.
[2] B.Eaglesfield and B.M. Phillips, *Liverpool Royal Infirmary Nurses' Training School 1862-1962* (Liverpool, 1962)

Chapter 8
Journey into Academia
Kate Morle

In 1960, in the lower sixth form of my high school, it was evident that the question, 'What are you going to do?' needed to be addressed. During one of my frequent sessions in the school library searching through the careers material, the nursing bro- chure for The Liverpool Royal Infirmary attracted my attention and prompted me to write to find out more.

Some thirty years later it is interesting to reflect upon the consequences of that letter. I had considered other careers, for example journalism or law, but my first and strongest wish at that time was to pursue a career in nursing. I had spent a prolonged period in hospital during my fourteenth year, when the strong smell of disinfected corridors, the crisp starched uniforms and the prospect of mixing with all sections of society had exerted a strong influence. My parents, though, were not enthusiastic about the idea that I should become a nurse. However a bargain was struck: I would remain at school to complete my 'A' level studies and then, should my chosen path prove too difficult physically or not match my expectations, I would look to univer- sity studies.

My interview with Miss Jackson, then Matron of Liverpool Royal Infirmary, was quite daunting, especially by comparison with today's more relaxed and less formal selection procedures. While it is hard to recall precise details of the interview, I can remember the approach to Miss Jackson's office: to reach the inner sanctum one had to walk through two outer offices. Miss Jackson was a statuesque figure, dressed in a dark navy serge dress, with a neat white collar. Her hat seemed to stand inches above her head and was immaculately starched and goffered. She sat behind an enormous desk throughout the course of the interview and impressed on me the demanding nature of nursing and the discipline associated with the profession. The interview was followed by a meeting with the home sister and a rather brief medical examination. I was offered a place for September 1962. By then I gained my 'A' levels so felt that I had allayed my parents' concern about possible alternatives should I wish to withdraw.

I have never regretted my decision. The experience has been rewarding; full of opportunities and challenges in an ever-changing environment. Throughout my training and on qualifying I found satisfaction in teaching and supervising; this was fortunate in that the apprenticeship system of training, whereby student nurses were expected to assume the dual roles of trainee nurse and employee simultaneously, was heavily reliant upon such interest. It was therefore hardly surprising that after I qualified I chose to apply to become an operating theatre sister, since such a position involved a firm commitment to teaching during the minimum of six weeks that student nurses spent in the operating theatres. This clinical placement required the sister to give lectures in all the many aspects of theatre work, and that she ensured that students gained experience in all technical aspects of the department as well as looking after patients, from the time they were wheeled into the suite until they left the recovery room.

My marriage in 1968 resulted in a move to Colchester. It was here that I was approached by the commanding officer of the Royal Army Medical Corps to establish a rolling programme for nurses to prepare them to work in a brand new purpose-built recovery unit. This was great fun although it was quite strange to be a civilian within the military environment and difficult to find the appropriate response to all the saluting encountered as one walked through the hospital premises.

Having enjoyed teaching in both Liverpool and Colchester, it was not surprising that when I returned to Liverpool I actively sought a teaching post with The United Liverpool Hospitals, as a Clinical Teacher based in The Royal Southern Hospital. After two years in post I felt that I needed further stimulation and a challenge, so became clinical teacher/tutor to the first cohort of nurses pursuing the degree of B.Sc. in Life Sciences combined with S.R.N. at the University of Liverpool. After a further period of five years, I began to explore possibilities for improving my own qualifications and discovered that the Department of Nursing at the University of Manchester was offering the opportunity for qualified nurses to pursue an M.Sc. in Nursing together with a Nurse Tutor qualification. After my experiences of academic nursing from 1971 - 76 I felt enthusiastic about developing my own professional profile and applied. Following two years of full-time study, I was successful in gaining an M.Sc., a Diploma in Advanced Nursing Studies and a Registered Nurse Teacher qualification. We were a small group of relatively mature students: two of us now hold chairs in nursing.

Despite my roots being deep within rural Cheshire, I always seemed to return 'home', which is what Liverpool was fast becoming. In 1978, having completed the course in Manchester, I became a lecturer in the University of Liverpool Nursing Studies Unit, in order to help to teach and develop the B.Sc. Life Sciences and S.R.N. course. This four-and-a-half year course represented a major innovation in nurse education in Liverpool.

Although it is only relatively recently that nursing has been taught at higher education level, the process by which it came to be established as an academic discipline began earlier than many might imagine. In Yorkshire at the turn of the century efforts were being made to develop a Certificate in Nursing which had greater standing than that provided by The General Infirmary at Leeds. It was suggested that the examinations for this certificate should be set and marked by the Yorkshire College (later to become the University of Leeds) and this proposal was supported by the college and the doctors of Leeds. The college involvement would have given the resulting certificate the standing of any of those granted by the regulated examining bodies and would, consequently, have been held in national standing in the same way as the qualifications given by universities to doctors and members of other professions. It was proposed that the practical examination of the nurses would be undertaken by a supervising committee of superintendent nurses or, if the Local Government

Board liked to appoint them, by nursing inspectors. While the scheme was well-supported, nothing seems to have come of it. It represented the most ambitious thinking about nurse education of its time, and if acted upon would have taken nursing into the general education system of the country at the beginning of the 20th century. Only now are the ideas raised during the early part of the century being advanced: by the end of the century, as a consequence of the education reforms embodied in Project 2000, nursing will assume full integration within the higher education sector. Presented to the profession for discussion in 1986, Project 2000 envisages that all colleges of nursing and midwifery will have links with institutions of higher education and that nursing qualifications will be at higher education diploma level.

From the 1860s, Liverpool made a significant contribution to the development of nursing, not only in the voluntary hospital setting but also in the workhouse infirmary and in the community. These developments were revolutionary and became the models for other initiatives throughout the country. It is interesting to note that the development of district nursing was the means locally whereby general nursing was actually transformed from that of a domestic servant level occupation to a vocation supported by an educational programme. All this was made possible through the philanthropy and foresight of William Rathbone. [1] The early developments provided an excellent infra-structure for the continued development of nursing. It was not surprising therefore that the initiatives within the profession in the late 1950s, to establish nursing within the higher education sector, were given serious consideration in Liverpool.

While Liverpool was not the first university in the country to establish a nursing course, it was not far behind the pioneers in this field. In May 1968 Mrs Betty Hoare, then Principal Nursing Officer (Education) with The United Liverpool Hospitals, presented the case to the Faculty of Science for an integrated degree course, a Bachelor of Science with a Registered General Nursing qualification, to be offered by the University of Liverpool. It was no secret that Miss Anne White, then Chief Nursing Officer of The United Liverpool Hospitals, regarded as a visionary by her contemporaries, had already made approaches to the Deans of the Faculties of Medicine and Science in an effort to establish a foothold for nursing within the university sector. The case presented by Mrs Hoare drew attention to the fact that 'the nursing profession in keeping abreast of developments in medicine needs to seek to improve standards of teaching and the quality of patient care continually'. It was recognised that there was a need to attract candidates of high calibre who could be prepared for leadership positions. The need to provide opportunities for some members of the nursing profession to have a greater than average knowledge of basic medical sciences, and an understanding of scientific principles and methods was acknowledged. In 1970 the Pro-Dean of the Faculty of Science wrote to the Vice-Chancellor outlining the contribution that the University could make to the education of nurses. Reference was made to the Integrated Human Biology and Nursing course offered at the University of Surrey and the feasibility of provision for a similar course in the newly initiated Life Sciences course. It was considered possible that prospective nursing and life sciences students could select courses which would provide an ideal scientific background for nursing. The proposed course was agreed in principle by both the Department of Health and Social Security and the General Nursing Council, and the Board of Governors of The United Liverpool Hospitals approved the provision of ten places in addition to their normal intake of student nurses.

In 1971 a course to enable suitable candidates to study for a Bachelor of Science degree and become registered nurses within a four-and-a-half year period commenced. It was classified as an experimental course, a term applied to nursing courses approved for registration which were completed in less than the standard three-year period normally required. It was considered that nurses prepared in such a way, having studied the biological sciences in depth, would bring a critical approach to nursing problems and be able to make a valuable contribution to the nursing service in clinical areas, in research, in administration and in teaching both in the community and in hospital. The course was based in accommodation within the Hospital College and supported by one senior nurse tutor and an assistant clinical nurse teacher. A working party made up of representatives from the Department of Health and Social Security, the General Nursing Council and the University supervised, managed and monitored the early development of the course.

Nationally, things were moving, too. In 1972 the Briggs Report recommended that between three and five per cent of the total national intake to nursing should be undergraduates or graduates. In 1974 the G.N.C. expressed the view that over a period of ten years it would wish to see approximately 1,000 of the total intake of nurses as graduates/undergraduates. Of these the Council suggested that forty-five per cent should be graduates who would take a shortened course in nursing, whilst fifty-five per cent would be undergraduates pursuing the associated courses, but that ultimately these courses would be replaced by degrees in nursing. It was at this time that the General Nursing Council suggested that Liverpool should consider the development of a degree in nursing.

The B.Sc./S.R.N. course produced good science graduates and competent nurses and continued to be offered until 1986. During the interim period the General Nursing Council had been replaced by the United Kingdom Central Council for Nursing, Midwifery and Health Visiting, with Boards of Nursing in each of the four countries - England; Northern Ireland; Scotland, and Wales - to undertake supervision of the standard and quality of nurse education.[2]

The United Kingdom had also become part of the European Community and the shortened fast track integrated course in nursing offered by this University did not meet the requirements in hours of time spent on a nursing course as agreed throughout the Community. Part of the problem lay in the numbers of hours allocated to purely nursing studies, but that apart, there remained increasing professional pressure to develop degrees in nursing as opposed to integrated degrees. It was as a consequence of discussions with The English National Board in 1986 that it was decided that the B.Sc./S.R.N. should no longer be offered.

The position of nursing in this University at that time was somewhat fragmented. The Nursing Studies Unit, based in the

Faculty of Science, had the responsibility for the B.Sc./S.R.N. course. The Health Visiting course was based in the Department of Community Health in the Faculty of Medicine. The Community Nurse Education Centre was with the Liverpool Health Authority in the Liverpool School of Nursing and was required to seek relocation in higher education by 1988 if the courses offered were to be approved. Concurrently, the discussion papers in circulation concerning nurse educational reform were strongly recommending links between schools of nursing and higher education. Following discussions with all parties concerned, and in particular as a result of the drive, support and enthusiasm of Professor Frank Harris, then Dean of the Faculty of Medicine, the Department of Nursing, which by then incorporated the former Nursing Studies Unit, Health Visiting and Community Nursing, was formally established in the Faculty of Medicine in 1987. The major thrust of activity during 1987/88 was to develop a Bachelor of Nursing degree for approval by the professional bodies and validated by the University of Liverpool; it was proposed that it would be made available to candidates for the academic year commencing October 1988. Negotiations with Liverpool Health Authority were successful in ensuring places for a maximum of twenty-five undergraduate nurses. Thus, a course offering a Bachelor of Nursing with Honours degree, incorporating first level registration as a nurse (Registered General Nurse, R.G.N.) and one further certificate in Health Visiting, or District Nursing or Clinical Nursing research, commenced in 1988.

During this time my 'title' within the University changed many times. 1986 saw me as lecturer within the Nursing Studies Unit. In 1987, prior to the resignation of Director of the Unit, my title was changed to Assistant Director of the Nursing Studies Unit and later that year I was appointed Acting Head of the Department of Nursing. In 1987 a Chair of Nursing was created. It was after much soul-searching that I applied for the post, handing in my application on the closing date. It had been a very hard year bringing teams together to work in unison on a joint venture within a very tight time schedule. The Chair Selection Committee met in April 1988. It was with some trepidation that I

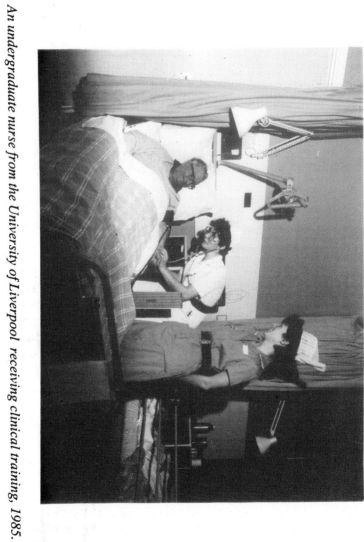

An undergraduate nurse from the University of Liverpool receiving clinical training, 1985.

answered the telephone at home that evening to confirm with the Vice-Chancellor, Professor Graeme Davies, my willingness to accept appointment to the first Chair of Nursing in the University of Liverpool.

At the time of taking up my appointment in May 1988, the department offered other nursing courses. These included Certificates in Health Visiting, District Nursing, a Practice Nurse Course and a Family Planning Course. Since that time the certificate courses in Health Visiting and District Nursing have been revalidated at Diploma Level and an M.Sc. in Nursing has also been validated: the first students enrolled in October 1991. Furthermore, a working group has submitted for validation a Diploma in Professional Studies (Nursing) which leads to a degree in Professional Studies (Nursing). This is a modular course which offers credit accumulation opportunities and is likely to be attractive to other professional disciplines apart from nursing.

Recently a Research and Development Unit was established in the department. The central focus of current research concerns clinical decision-making in selected situations and between different professional groups. This is an extremely active unit and has been successful in gaining substantial research funds. Currently there are approximately seven research students and assistants, together with a growing number of full- and part-time Ph.D. students.

The department serves as a resource unit for health service colleagues, facilitating their skills in research methods and application; the latter function is particularly significant in increasing research-based nursing practice.

Initially the development of departments of nursing, and the provision of degrees either in nursing or associated with other degree subjects, could in many ways be regarded as an act of faith and confidence since it was not for some considerable time that it was possible to review the impact of graduates upon the profession. Whilst the perpetual problems dogging nursing

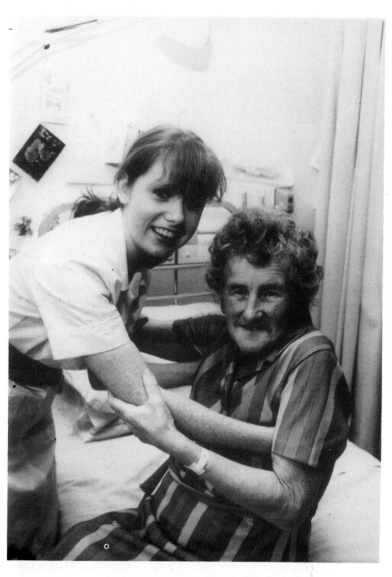

An undergraduate nurse from the Department of Nursing, the
University of Liverpool, assisting a patient, 1992.

appear to be related to recruitment, retention and wastage, research has revealed a significantly lower drop-out rate from universities compared with schools of nursing; a higher proportion of graduates remain in nursing for longer periods than non-graduate nurses, and, to date, recruitment targets have been readily met. Differences emerge between graduates and other trained nurses when analyzing career patterns, chosen specialities and participation in continuing education. Two thirds of graduates choose to remain in jobs which involve patient care. This striking trend is reflected in their choice of speciality. There are more who opt for psychiatry, care of the elderly, intensive care and community nursing than is found in any average group of registered nurses. At least two thirds also choose to take another post-registration course, usually after a period of one or two years general nursing, during which time they consolidate their skills. The above average representation of graduates choosing care of the elderly is particularly noteworthy, in view of the increasing numbers of elderly in our society. 'Cinderella' areas such as these are seen to be attractive to graduates, who recognise opportunities to become more independent in their practice and to improve standards of care.

So far as clinical skills are concerned, observation and research work indicate that graduates make a substantially greater contribution to certain aspects of care. Most university courses emphasise psychological care and communication skills - this results in improved care, both in preventing unnecessary morbidity as a consequence of stress and in enhanced support for those recovering from illness or coping with chronic disorders. There are indications that graduates spend longer engaged in direct patient care than other trained staff prepared in courses during which longer, more concentrated, periods of training are spent as members of the workforce.

The significant contribution to developments in nursing made by the university nursing departments is in the area of nursing research. No group can be considered truly professional unless there is an established scientific basis to their practice. Within a relatively short period, nursing research has provided an increased understanding of issues in clinical nursing practice. Research studies have also been undertaken in the fields of nursing education and nurse management. The extent of this activity is commendable when judged against the relatively short period which nurses in the United Kingdom have had to acquire the requisite research techniques. Progressively there has been growing concern over the widening gap between higher education and clinical nursing, as evidenced by the growing volume of nursing research which is under-utilised. The proposals to increase the graduate nurse population, through educational reform and by increasing the number of undergraduate places, are recognised as the means of improving the situation.

It is apparent that departments of nursing will continue to hold the major responsibility for enabling critical evaluation of existing research findings, not only through replication of existing research studies, since many of these have involved relatively small samples, but also through innovative research into nursing practice. Departments of nursing will continue to facilitate the dissemination of research relative to nursing, progressively developing the theory underpinning the practice of nursing. In a climate in which the emphasis is increasingly upon effectiveness and efficiency within the clinical setting these responsibilities are of crucial significance. Furthermore, the constant demands and challenges as changes present themselves both within higher education and the health service, require increasingly imaginative and innovative responses in order to advance the continued development of the profession of nursing.

During a span of little more than thirty years nursing education has undergone considerable change and continues to evolve, ensuring that the nursing profession responds to the needs and expectations of practitioners and recipients of care. My own personal and professional development is representative of precisely those changes as they have occurred. I have been fortunate to have been able to take opportunities as they have arisen and to have had support and encouragement from many people.

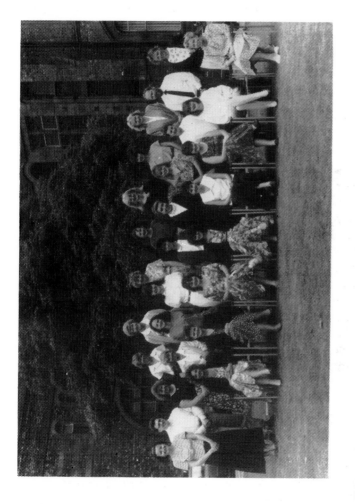

Bachelor of Nursing graduands, University of Liverpool, Summer 1992, together with some members of the staff of the University Department of Nursing.

Notes

[1] See Gwen Hardy, *William Rathbone and the Early History of District Nursing* (Ormskirk, 1981)

[2] These boards are The English National Board for Nursing, Midwifery and Health Visiting; The Welsh National Board for Nursing, Midwifery and Health Visiting; The National Board for Nursing, Midwifery and Health Visiting for Scotland; and The National Board for Nursing, Midwifery and Health Visiting for Northern Ireland.

Chapter 9

Sources for the History of Nursing
in Liverpool
Adrian Allan

Introduction

A   Secondary sources

B   Primary sources

1. General

2. Public Record Office

3. Department of Manuscripts, The British Library

4. Contemporary Medical Archives Centre

5. National Film and Television Archive

6. Royal College of Obstetricians and Gynaecologists

7. Lancashire Record Office

8. Charity Commission

9. Liverpool Health Authority

10. Liverpool Record Office and Local History Library

11. Merseyside Record Office

12. North West Film Archive

13. Special Collections Department, Sydney Jones Library, University of Liverpool

14. University Archives, Liverpool

15. Records which have not been deposited in a record office, etc.

16. Artefacts

Introduction

This chapter aims to introduce some of the principal secondary and primary sources for the history of nursing in Liverpool. It should be emphasised that in the case of both the library and the record repository, accessions of publications and records are constantly being received whereby any 'guide' is bound to be out-of-date to some degree: the researcher thus needs to seek information on more recent accessions (some of which may not become immediately available for research until they have been listed or catalogued). A more extensive list of the primary sources (with their individual record office references) together with a full introduction to the secondary sources for the history of nursing in both Liverpool and its region has been compiled by the author of this chapter and copies may be purchased upon application to him at the University of Liverpool Archives.

A useful introduction to historical research in the context of nursing history is provided by Anne Marie Rafferty in chapter 18, 'Historical Research', in Desmond F.S. Cormack (ed.), *The Research Process in Nursing* (Oxford, 2nd ed., 1991). She has also contributed chapter 2, 'Historical Perspectives', to Kate Robinson and Barbara Vaughan (eds.), *Knowledge for Nursing Practice* (Oxford, 1992).

A   Secondary sources

The published source material for the history of nursing basically comprises both (a) the contemporary publications of the period being studied and (b) the growing number of books, journal articles and theses on various aspects of the history of nursing which have been published over the last thirty years.

The contemporary publications include national journals (including *The Nursing Times,* 1905 onwards); reports of government-appointed committees (such as that of the Royal Commission on the Poor Laws, 1909); other reports (for instance the annual reports of Medical Officers of Health); national directories (such as *Burdett's Hospital Annual*, 1890-93 and its successor, the annual *Burdett's Hospitals and Charities*, 1894-1930); local directories (including Gore's, later Kelly's, Liverpool Directory for the years 1766 onwards); and the invaluable files of the local press (such as the *Liverpool General Advertiser*, later entitled *Gore's General Advertiser*, which was published 1765-1876) with their full reports on the meetings of local authorities, nursing associations, etc.

Liverpool Central Libraries, William Brown Street, holds copies of a number of these published sources (in the form of microfilm copies in the case of the local directories and local press files), which may be freely consulted. The sheaf catalogue to the Local History Library, Liverpool Central Libraries, alone provides references to over 50 publications (books and articles, annual reports, brochures, etc.) on the subject of nursing in Liverpool.

For information (including names, addresses and opening hours) about library and information services in Merseyside, including academic libraries and medical and nursing libraries in the region, see T.W. Scragg (compiler), *Merseyside Directory of Reference and Information Services* (7th ed., 1992), available from Knowsley Central Library, Derby Road, Huyton, L36 9UJ.

B. Primary sources

1. General

A useful introduction to sources generally is provided by Janet Foster and Julia Sheppard in their chapter on 'Archives and the History of Nursing' in Celia Davies (ed.), *Rewriting Nursing History* (London, 1980). Rather than providing an indication of the variety of primary sources (ranging from the records of schools of nursing to those of nursing associations and from written records to visual and oral records), this present chapter provides summary notes about the many such records as relate to Liverpool as are to be found in both national and local record repositories and elsewhere. As already mentioned in the Introduction to this chapter, extensive lists of these records are available upon application.

Invaluable guides to record repositories, national and local, are provided by the following:-

Janet Foster and Julia Sheppard, *British Archives: A Guide to Archive Resources in the United Kingdom* (London, 2nd ed., 1989); reference copies of this substantial work should be found in the principal local libraries and in local record offices.

Margaret Procter (compiler), *Archives on Merseyside : A Guide to Local Repositories* (2nd ed., 1992); copies available from Merseyside Record Office, 4th floor, Cunard Building, Pier Head, Liverpool, L3 1EG.

A survey of hospital archives (and artefacts) within Mersey Regional Health Authority's area (Merseyside and Cheshire) was undertaken in 1981-82 by the Health Records Survey team based at the University Archives, Liverpool. In addition, surveys were made of the holdings of some local libraries (including that of the Liverpool Medical Institution, which holds copies of the annual reports of the Liverpool Royal Infirmary Nurses Training School Nurses League,

116

for 1935-37 and 1939-64, besides local medical journals, etc.) The resultant lists were supplied to the relevant health authorities, hospitals and local record offices. Unfortunately, not all the records surveyed (which included registers of nurses) have as yet been deposited in the appropriate local record office. Copies of the lists may be seen at the University Archives.

2. **Public Record Office**
   Ruskin Avenue, Kew, Richmond, Surrey, TW9 4DU

A very useful introduction to relevant sources in the PRO, prefaced by historical introductions, is the PRO's *Records Information* No.113: *Civilian Nurses and Nursing Services: Record Sources in the Public Record Office* (1990), copies of which are obtainable (free of charge) upon application to the PRO. It should be noted that most of such records are generally closed to access for 30 years after the date of the file etc. in question.

Amongst records in the PRO of particular value are those of:-

(a) the *General Nursing Council* (established 1919, dissolved 1979).

   Includes the correspondence and papers of the Liverpool Area Nurse Training Committee, 1951-70; correspondence with Miss Mary Jones, a GNC member, and copies of her reports on Liverpool hospitals, 1932-59; hospital inspectors' reports and papers covering almost all hospitals (and hospital schools of nursing) in the region, 1936-79; correspondence and papers re nurse training and nurse training schools in the region, 1920-83; and correspondence etc. re degree courses in nursing, etc. at the University of Liverpool, Liverpool Polytechnic, and Sefton School of Nursing, 1967-83.

117

(b) the *Central Midwives Board* (1902-83)

> Includes correspondence with Liverpool Royal Hospital, 1947-52, papers re experimental training scheme at Liverpool, 1949-54, and reports on training hospitals in the region, 1938-80.

(c) the (unpublished) *Public Health Surveys,* conducted by the Ministry of Health staff, which refer to provision of nurses in hospitals, nurse training, nursing associations and other voluntary bodies; the files which cover Liverpool date from 1932-39.

(d) the *Queen's Institute of District Nursing,* comprising correspondence with and annual reports on county and district nursing associations made by the Institute's Inspectors in the Liverpool region, 1892-1948.

Census Enumerators' Schedules

Mention should also be made of the Census Enumerators' Schedules for 1841,1851,1861,1871,1881, and 1891 which the Public Record Office holds. Microfilm copies (not the originals) may be inspected at the PRO's Chancery Lane office, London, WC2. The microfilm unit of Liverpool Central Libraries (William Brown Street) holds microfilm copies of the Schedules covering Liverpool and surrounding districts (i.e. Prescot, Toxteth Park, etc.) for all six censuses (1841-91). The Schedules cover not only individual houses, etc., but also hospitals, asylums, workhouses, nurses' homes, etc., recording those resident at the time the census was taken.

3. **Department of Manuscripts, The British Library**
Great Russell Street, London, WC1B 3DG

Amongst the holdings of the Department are the correspondence and papers of Florence Nightingale (1820-1910). They include (a) her correspondence etc. with Agnes E. Jones,

Lady Superintendent of Liverpool Workhouse Infirmary, 1861-68; (b) her correspondence with Mr. William Rathbone, M.P., 1860-1902; and (c) typewritten copies of her letters to William Rathbone (from originals then in the Queen's Institute of District Nursing).

4. **Contemporary Medical Archives Centre**
    Wellcome Institute for the History of Medicine, 183 Euston Road, London, NW1 2BN

Brief descriptions of the holdings of the Centre are given in Julia Sheppard and Lesley Hall (compilers), *A Guide to the Contemporary Medical Archives Centre* (CMAC, Wellcome Institute for the History of Medicine, London, 1991).

The CMAC holds the majority of the older records of the Queen's Nursing Institute (ref. SA/QNI). These basically comprise those of the Institute of Nursing Sisters (minutes 1841-1939, register of nurses c.1840-c.1855) and the Queen Victoria Institute of Nursing (minutes, annual reports, and correspondence, 1898-c.1939), together with registers and rolls of Queen's Nurses, 1891-1969; registers and rolls of affiliated local associations, 1890-1939; federation and branch minutes and annual reports, 1890-1973; and a collection of letters, pamphlets, notes, etc. collected for Mary Stocks when she was writing *A Hundred Years of District Nursing* (1960). Amongst these QNI records are (a) some correspondence of William Rathbone the sixth and (b) minutes, correspondence, plans, summary history, etc. of the William Rathbone Staff College, Liverpool, 1940-70.

Amongst the QNI records some years ago (when in the custody of the QNI) were two volumes of reports written by Florence Lees, one of which, a report on district nursing in Liverpool, 1875, was later reported missing. Liverpool Record Office holds transcripts of both volumes which Mrs. Gwen Hardy made while they were held by the QNI.

5. **National Film and Television Archive**
British Film Institute, 21 Stephen Street, London, W1P 1PL

For a guide, see *National Film Archive Catalogue* (1965-80), volume 1 of which (1980) covers non-fiction films. Manchester Central Library holds a copy of this catalogue; neither the Liverpool City Libraries nor the University of Liverpool Library at present hold a copy of the volume covering non-fiction films. These films include:-

      1316   A record of the visit of HM Queen Mary to Fazakerley Hospital, Liverpool, 1915

6. **Royal College of Obstetricians and Gynaecologists**
27 Sussex Place, Regent's Park, London, NW1 4RG

Amongst the College's archives are two collections of the papers of Professor William Blair-Bell (1871-1936), Professor of Midwifery and Gynaecology at the University of Liverpool 1921-31 and first President of the College. They include the following (access by prior arrangement with the College Archivist):-

(a) Letters from patients or prospective patients of Blair-Bell re treatment for cancer and possible admission to a nursing home in Rodney Street, Liverpool, 1919-29, and other correspondence and papers re his professional and domestic life.

(b) Correspondence re Blair-Bell's practice in Liverpool (particularly the Nursing Home for Cancer Patients), and correspondence with the University of Liverpool and with tradesmen, 1922-31.

(c) Papers re private nursing home in Rodney Street.

7. **Lancashire Record Office**
   Bow Lane, Preston, PR1 2RE

   For a summary guide to the records deposited at the office up to and including 1989, see R. Sharpe France, *Guide to the Lancashire Record Office* (Lancashire County Council, 1985) and J.D. Martin (ed.), *Guide to the Lancashire Record Office: A Supplement* (Lancashire County Books, 1992).

   Amongst the deposited records are the minutes, reports, and correspondence of Garston (later Garston and Grassendale) District Nursing Association, 1873-1951, ref. DDX 1033.

8. **Charity Commission**
   5th floor, Graeme House, Derby Square, Liverpool, L2 7SB

   The Liverpool office of the Charity Commission covers the north of England and also Wales. Copies of governing instruments and annual reports and accounts for charities in the region may be found on Central Register files (most recent records) and on Charitable Trust files (earlier records), both kept at the Liverpool office. Some of these files are open to public inspection.

   Amongst the files is one, Registration no. 223242, re the Walter Harding Treats Trust (which funded theatre parties, Llandudno steamer outings, a hospitals tennis tournament, etc. for nursing staff in Liverpool and Wirral): it comprises copies of the will of Walter Harding (d.1936), declaration of trust of the charity (1937), and accounts for 1961-86 (incomplete series). The beneficiaries of the will included individual nursing staff and hospitals; the will permitted Harding's trustees to sell The Claremont Nursing Home, Birkenhead (which he owned) at a discount to its matron, Miss Bullock.

9. **Liverpool Health Authority**

The Liverpool Health Authority has retained a large quantity of non-current records, including (a) a register of lying-in homes, later of nursing homes, 1922-81 (details number and qualifications of nursing staff, etc.), (b) minutes and papers of Liverpool Area Nursing and Midwifery Committee, 1974-82, and (c) files of correspondence etc. re Woolton Manor Nurse Education Centre, nursing centres, nursing homes, nursing services, nurses homes and accommodation, and the Mersey Regional Nurse Training Committee, 1973-88. Enquiries should be addressed to the Liverpool Health Authority, 1st floor, 8 Mathew Street, Liverpool, L2 6RE.

10. **Liverpool Record Office and Local History Library**
Central Libraries, William Brown Street, Liverpool, L3 8EW

For a guide to the records (and publications) relating to public health (including hospital archives) held by the Office, see Margaret Procter (ed.), *Public Health on Merseyside : A Guide to Sources* (Merseyside Archives Liaison Group, Liverpool, 1991), copies of which may be purchased at Liverpool Record Office (and other local record offices on Merseyside). The records of Liverpool City Council's Hospitals and Port Health Committee (which are summarily listed in the *Guide*) include the minutes of the Special Sub-Committee with regard to nurses' uniforms, 1936-37, which are referred to in ch.2.

Amongst the records of Liverpool hospitals which have been deposited and which are relevant are the following. The general reference for the Record Office's hospital record holdings is 614.

(a)   *Alder Hey Children's Hospital*: Nursing Sub-Committee and Nurses' Education Committee minutes 1948-52, 1957-71, and photographs of staff, etc.

(b)   *David Lewis Northern Hospital:* Nursing Committee minutes, 1930-34; valuation of Nurses' Home furniture and equipment, 1940; Hospital's Nurses' League annual report, etc., 1959; forms for the employment of hospital nurses in private families, n.d.

(c)   *Hahnemann Hospital:* nursing medals, 1887.

(d)   *Liverpool Eye and Ear Infirmary*, later the *Liverpool Ear, Nose and Throat Infirmary:* Probationer Nurses' Record Book, 1926-52.

(e)   *Liverpool Maternity Hospital:* Report book of the Ladies' Charity (reports on individual cases), 1826-69; newscuttings, correspondence, etc. re dispute between doctors and matron, 1895-6; minutes of Teaching [of pupil midwives] Committee, 1945-49; register and lists of nursing staff, 1906-37, c.1952-55; Nurses Home inventory, 1956; programmes of courses, 1932-33; brochure on hospital's School of Midwifery, 1962.

(f)   *Liverpool Royal Infirmary:* Training School and Home for Nurses Committee, later the Nursing Committee, minutes 1874-1938; annual reports of the Training School and Home for Nurses for 1862-1937; annual reports of matrons of the Royal Liverpool United Hospital, 1938-47; annual reports of the Training School Nurses' League, 1935-46, 1953, and 1955-56; matron's reports, 1917-38, and petty cash book 1932-48; nursing staff wage books, 1882-1921, and register of donations, 1932-52, and related papers; rules and regulations for nurses, etc., 1892-1949; registers of nursing staff and students, 1862-1957; papers re probationer nurses and nursing staff, 1869-1921; nurses' examination papers and record of results, 1908-18; correspondence re nursing and individual nurses, 1858-1941; registers of stock of linen, hardware etc., in wards, etc., 1934-56; visitors' book of the United Liverpool Hospitals' Nurses' Preliminary Training School, Woolton Manor, 1954-66; photographs etc. of nursing staff, wards, PTS and its staff and students, nurses' home and furnishings, etc., [1880]-[?1970s]; scrap books of press cuttings, programmes, and photographs and loose press cuttings re nurses, Nurses' Home, Nurses' Training School, etc., 1896-1963; programmes of Red Rose Balls, opening of new Nurses' Home, Cathedral services, etc., 1921-54; 'Nurses' Purse' and 'Sisters' Purse' presented to HRH the Duchess of York on the opening of the new Nurses' Home, 1923.

(g)   *Liverpool Stanley Hospital:* correspondence, regulations, and reports re nursing, nursing staff, etc., 1949-64.

(h)   *Royal Liverpool Children's Hospital:* Nursing Committee minutes 1945-48; Matron's Report Book, 1935-49; Registers of nurses, 1910-57; Register of nursery nurses course, 1942-43.

(i)   *Royal Southern Hospital:* Nursing Committee minutes, 1901-43; Student Nurses' Unit Committee minutes, 1942-46; annual reports of hospital's Nursing Institution, 1887-1907; nurses registers and record books, 1873-1952; Nursing Certificates, 1960s; Nurses' League Minutes, 1957-80 and Journals, 1958-79; transcript of letters from Florence Nightingale to William Rathbone the sixth, (1864)-(1900); centenary papers, 1971-2, including correspondence with Nurses' League; albums of photographs of nurses, wards, etc., of both this hospital and also the Children's Infirmary, Myrtle Street and West Kirby Children's Convalescent Home, [c.1900]-1960; and Bon Voyage, organ of the Nurses' Social Club, 1940.

124

(j)   *St. Paul's Eye Hospital:* Nursing registers, etc.
        were deposited in the Record Office in 1992.

        (Amongst the records which the University Ar-
        chives Health Records Survey team listed in 1981
        as being at the hospital were registers of nursing
        staff, 1923-55; staff attendance register, 1948-58;
        list of annual salaries of nursing and auxiliary staff,
        1915-16; and reports of the Matron to the Hospital
        Committee, 1942-70, besides annual reports of the
        hospital, 1873-1947, etc.)

(k)   *Sefton General Hospital:* 5 photographs of scenes
        in male and female wards.

        (A large quantity of records of the hospital have
        been more recently deposited with the Record Of-
        fice: they may include some of the 30-odd volumes
        of registers of nursing staff, matron's report book,
        etc., 1906-55, which were recorded as being at the
        hospital in 1981).

(l)   *United Liverpool Hospitals*, etc: Handbooks of
        nurse and midwifery training schools and of Liver-
        pool Queen Victoria District Nursing Association,
        c.1910-[?1950s]; nursing certificates, 1911, ?1940s;
        photographs of nurses, nurses training, nurses' ac-
        commodation, etc., [c.1910]-1970s, also of 19th
        century and modern toys at Heswall Children's
        Hospital; press report on public meeting to consider
        establishing a Training School and Home for Nurses,
        (1862); papers (correspondence, photographs, press
        cuttings, programmes, badges, etc.) of Miss Mary
        Jones (Matron, Liverpool Royal Infirmary, 1925-
        47), 1908-71.

        (see full list by University Archives' Health Records
        Survey Team, 1982)

(m) *United Liverpool Hospitals:* monthly statistics of staff and establishments of constituent hospitals, 1969 (ref. Acc.4856).

(n) *Women's Hospital, Catherine Street:* expenditure analysis book (including nursing salaries, dressings, etc.), 1932-37.

The relative preponderance amongst the surviving records of hospitals of the registers of nursing staff and students will be noted in the above listing and in the lists of records in the other local record offices, and calls for a brief comment. To some degree, the nature of the information recorded in these registers varies from one hospital to another, but the case of those of Liverpool Royal Infirmary illustrates the range of the information that may be recorded (and reveals its obvious considerable research potential). For instance, the first volume of the Infirmary's Register of Probationer Nurses, 1862-76, records not only name, age and date of appointment of each probationer, but also her marital status, by whom she was recommended, the names of the nurses under whom she served, her religion, the nature of her duties, details of the work she carried out (dressings, applying leeches, enemas, bandaging, making beds, sick cooking, etc.), and comments on her record of punctuality, etc. and on her sobriety, honesty, and truthfulness during her probationary period.

Amongst the records of associations, societies and individuals which the Record Office holds are:-

(a) *Liverpool Queen Victoria District Nursing Association* (formed in 1898), ref. Acc.3066: press cuttings, programmes, photographs, etc., 1896-1970s, 1960-75; correspondence and financial papers, 1902-35; transcript of reports read at Executive Committee, also accounts, register of nurses, statistics of cases nursed, etc., 1899-1903; letters of William Rathbone re district nursing and Central

Nurses' Home, 1890-98, and copy of correspondence of Florence Nightingale with him, (1862)-(1885); minutes of meetings of [benefactors of] a District Nurses Home, Edge Hill, 1897-1923; inventory of furnishings at a District Nurses Home [early 20th century]; notes, plans, and copies of articles etc. re Central Home (later Staff College), 1898-1974; correspondence, programme, circulars etc. re Jubileē Congress of District Nursing at Liverpool, 1909; Notes on district nursing, duties of nurses, etc., [?late 19th century - c.1910]; correspondence, appeal brochure etc. re Florence Nightingale Memorial, Liverpool, 1909-11; account of nursing in Liverpool schools, [?c.1909]; reports of Queen Victoria's Jubilee Institute for Nurses' inspection of nursing associations (including Cheshire County Nursing Association and Birkenhead District Nursing Society) and homes, 1908-09.

(b)   *Woolton and District Nursing Society* (formed in 1879), ref. 362 WOO: Committee minutes 1895-8, 1918-50, 1964; correspondence, etc. re charities, Jubilee Nursing Trust, etc., 1899-1963; annual reports, 1880-1947, and accounts, 1948-55; appeal for subscriptions and donations, 1879; also annual report of Garston and Grassendale District Nursing Association, 1923.

(c)   Dr. Thomas H. Bickerton's collections of papers, upon which was based his *A Medical History of Liverpool ... to the year 1920* (1936), include sections on Midwifery and on Nurses (ref. 942 BIC 9-10).

(d)   Photocopies of letters from Florence Nightingale re Agnes Jones [later Matron of Liverpool Workhouse Infirmary] and re proposed public infirmaries in Liverpool, (1864) (ref. 920 AUT).

(e)   West Derby Union Institutions Liverpool Training
       Schools for Nurses: Nurses Certificate awarded to
       Miss I.L. Pickering, 1919 (ref. Acc. 4751).

(f)   Papers of Mary C. Davies (ref. Acc. 4886): notes on
       lectures on General Nursing etc. at the David Lewis
       Northern Hospital, examination papers, register of
       midwifery cases (while at Smithdown Road Hospi-
       tal), and press cuttings, 1931-37.

(g)   Royal Liverpool Hospital Nurses' League: minutes
       and miscellaneous papers, 1973-92 (ref. Acc. 4901).

(h)   List of articles required by Probationer Nurses,
       Brownlow Hill Institution Infirmary and photo-
       graphs of Matron, nursing staff and resident doctors
       of the Infirmary, c.1926 (ref. Acc. 3529).

11. **Merseyside Record Office**
    4th floor, Cunard Building, Pier Head, Liverpool, L3 1EG

    The Record Office holds copies of the published annual
    reports and accounts of a number of charities which were
    submitted to the Charity Commission (ref. 364 CHC). They
    include:-

(a)   Nursing Associations, etc. - Garston and Grassendale
       District Nursing Association (accounts, 1945, an-
       nual reports, 1943-44, 1946); Liverpool Queen
       Victoria District Nursing Association (annual re-
       ports, 1927, 1931-32); Welsford Nurses' Relief
       Fund (Liverpool) (accounts, 1927-32); and Woolton
       and District Nursing Society (incomplete set of
       accounts, 1902-26, and annual reports, 1922-47).

(b)   Eight individual voluntary hospitals in Liverpool -
       annual reports covering the period 1904-46.

It is intended to deposit with the Record Office the tape-recorded interviews of retired nurses which Mrs. Frances Trees has been making (1991 onwards), together with the associated documentation. Copies of these tapes will also be made available to the National Museums and Galleries on Merseyside and to the Royal College of Nursing Archives.

12. **North West Film Archive**
The Manchester Metropolitan University, Minshull House, 47-49 Chorlton Street, Manchester, M1 3EU.

Amongst the Archive's holdings are films of:-

(a)   Liverpool Invalid Children's Association Child Welfare Centre, c.1916, ref. 35.

(scenes at the Central Office, Liverpool and at Leasowe Hospital, Wirral)

(b)   Gaumont Graphic Newsreel, 1927-32, including opening [in 1932] of the Liverpool and Samaritan Hospital for Women [the Women's Hospital, Catharine Street, Liverpool], ref. 110.

13. **Special Collections Department,**
Sydney Jones Library, University of Liverpool
P.O. Box 147, Liverpool, L69 3BX

Amongst the Rathbone family papers are (a) correspondence and papers on District Nursing, 1867-1911, consisting chiefly of letters from William Rathbone the sixth to various correspondents, 1891, 1894-95 (ref. Rathbone Papers ix.6.66-100), and (b) letters to William Rathbone the sixth from Florence Nightingale, 1890-1902 (Rathbone Papers ix.7.184-86).

The Department also holds a typescript transcript of letters from Florence Nightingale to William Rathbone the sixth, 1864-1900 (ref. MS.4.1), and a letter from the former to the latter, 1900 (ref. MS.3.52 (195)).

14. University Archives, Liverpool
Harold Cohen Library, P.O. Box 147, Liverpool, L69 3BX

The University Archives holds the archives of the Faculty of Medicine and of individual departments of the Faculty (which include the Department of Nursing), together with records deposited by medical graduates, etc. Amongst the records are:-

(a)   Reminiscences of Dr. William S. Paget-Tomlinson, referring to his period as a student at the Liverpool Royal Infirmary School of Medicine (1866-70) and subsequently, which refers to the Practical Midwifery course (1868-9), etc. (ref. D.40/15)

(b)   Photocopy of recollections of medical career in Liverpool (including period at Medical School) and later in Birkenhead of Dr. Sidney B. Herd (b.1899), including an account of Obstetrics and Gynaecology in Liverpool (particularly the Domiciliary Midwifery Association of Liverpool Maternity Hospital) and his role (as a Gynaecologist) assisting successive Professors, etc; includes references to nursing staff of Liverpool Royal Infirmary, Red Rose Ball, etc. (ref. D.87)

(c)   Account books of Rodney House Nursing Home and 48 Rodney Street, Liverpool (Private Patients Nursing Home directed by Professor W. Blair-Bell), 1926-32 (ref. D.106/9)

(d)   Colour film of Woolton Preliminary Training School for Nurses, Liverpool, and of its official opening, March 1954, taken by Dr. Robert R. Hughes (ref. D.352/8)

(e)   Photographs taken by Dr. Frank Neubert as a medical student at Liverpool, 1929-39, include a number of individual and group photographs of members of the nursing staff of Liverpool Maternity Hospital, Liverpool Royal Infirmary, Liverpool Women's Hospital, Walton Hospital, and the David Lewis Northern Hospital (ref. D.361)

(f)   Papers of Mrs. Gwyneth Sanderson (née Owen), formerly a Sister at Liverpool Royal Infirmary, including copies of photographs of nurses singing carols at the Infirmary and nurses on the steps of Liverpool Cathedral [c.1939, 1941]; copies of the journals of The United Liverpool Hospitals' Nurses' League (later The Royal Liverpool Hospital Nurses' League) for 1974-79 and 1986; and recollections and tape-recorded recollections of her nursing career and of her late husband, Dr. Gerard Sanderson, 1987 (ref. D.421)

(g)   A note on the dress of surgeons working in the Liverpool Royal Infirmary by Mr. Clifford Brewer, FRCS, 1990; refers to the duties of theatre nursing staff (ref. D.478)

(h)   Correspondence, agenda papers, reports, and copies of press cuttings and relevant publications re the proposed University of Liverpool B.Sc./S.R.N. course (which started in September 1971), 1966-79 (ref. A.105/1-3)

(i)   Agenda papers of meetings of the University of Liverpool Nursing Studies Unit, later of the Department of Nursing's General Nursing Section, and related papers, 1982-87 (ref. A.105/4)

(j)   Copies of photographs of Professor John Hay (Professor of Medicine, 1924-34) together with nursing staff of Liverpool Royal Infirmary, the operating theatre and staff of the Infirmary, Miss Mary Jones (Matron), and others, (c.1896-97), (1933-34), ([?1930s]); and photographs of Professor Hay's cartoon sketches of Miss Mary Jones, n.d. (ref. D.98/2)

15. Records which have not been deposited in a record office, etc.

Besides the records of hospitals which have not, as yet, been deposited in local record offices, there are other records relating to the history of nursing which have likewise not been deposited. They include:-

In the custody of the *Department of Obstetrics and Gynaecology, University of Liverpool:* copies of the annual reports of the Ladies Charity and Lying-in-Hospital (later the Liverpool Maternity Hospital and Ladies Charity) for 1883-1921; 'Practical Midwifery: Rules for Students': regulations, reports, etc., 1895-1906; and correspondence of Professors Paterson and Briggs re practical midwifery element of Medical School's course, 1893-1914.

16. Artefacts

In some cases artefacts (such as nursing badges and medals) have been deposited together with the archives in local record offices, and some are referred to in the above lists of holdings of Liverpool Record Office. In some other cases, such objects have sometimes been deposited with a museum or art gallery.

The Department of Regional History, National Museums and Galleries on Merseyside, (at the Merseyside Maritime Museum, Albert Dock, Liverpool) has a growing collection of nursing artefacts, including costume, badges, memorial plaques, nursing certificates and some nursing equipment. The Department has also a considerable number of negatives of images related to the nursing profession in Liverpool, such as photographs, prints and book illustrations. This collection is available to researchers.

The University of Liverpool Art Collections include the Liverpool Royal Infirmary gold medal presented to the top nursing examinee in 1930, and the silver rose bowl presented by the Infirmary's Medical Board to the retiring Matron in 1948. Other artefacts, principally emanating from hospitals, are believed to have been deposited in other museums and collections in the region, besides those objects which have been deposited with national collections (especially The Wellcome Museum of the History of Medicine, a part of the National Museum of Science and Industry, South Kensington, London).

More broadly, one might argue that the records of nursing are not only to be found in the record office, library, and museum (and in private custody), but also in the recollections of those who have experienced nursing (whether as practitioner or as patient), and in the design and use of the buildings (hospitals, nursing homes, etc.) with which they have been associated.

SELECT BIBLIOGRAPHY

Brian Abel-Smith *A History of the Nursing Profession* (London, 1960)
The Hospitals, 1800-1948: A Study in Social Administration in England and Wales (London, 1964)

Monica E. Baly *Nursing and Social Change* (2nd edition, London, 1980)
Florence Nightingale and the Nursing Legacy (London, 1986)

'The Briggs Report' *Report of the Committee on Nursing* (Chairman: Professor Asa Briggs) (Cmnd 5115, H.M.S.O., London, 1972)

Helen Cohen *The Nurse's Quest for a Professional Identity* (California, 1981)

Celia Davies (ed.) *Rewriting Nursing History* (London, 1980)

Robert Dingwall,
Anne Marie Rafferty and
Charles Webster *An Introduction to the Social History of Nursing* (London, 1988)

B. Eaglesfield and
B. M. Phillips *Liverpool Royal Infirmary Nurses' Training School 1862-1962* (Liverpool, 1962)

Gwen Hardy *William Rathbone and the Early History of District Nursing* (Ormskirk, 1981)

Christopher Maggs *The Origins of General Nursing* (London, 1983)

Patricia Owens and
Howard Glennerster *Nursing in Conflict* (Basingstoke, 1990)

Mary Stocks *A Hundred Years of District Nursing* (London, 1960)

Charles Webster	*The Health Services since the War* vol.I, *Problems of health care. The National Health Service before 1957* (London, 1988)
Rosemary White	*Social Change and the Development of the Nursing Profession: A Study of the Poor Law Nursing Service, 1848-1948* (London, 1978) *The Effects of the NHS on the Nursing Profession, 1948 - 1961* (London, 1985) *Political Issues in Nursing,* vols.1&3 (London, 1985 & 1988)

Index

G

J

K

L

R

S

T

U

V

W

L. LANE